Dramatic Weight Loss Using BDSM – Huge Bonus Edition – 10 eBooks in One!

By Phil G.

Copyright (C) 2013

ISBN-13: 978-1492729624
ISBN-10: 1492729620

Erotic BDSM Books - Your Erotic BDSM Book Publisher
EroticBDSMbooks.com

Included also are nine free bonus books (making this book a $69.50 value!) Your books are presented in this order:

Other Books by EroticBDSMbooks.com Include:

*The Absolutely Essential Book of BDSM and S&M Rules
*Things To Do During 3 Hours of Sex; A Step-by-step Guide
*Playtime At The Dom Den; A Step-by-step Guide
*The Absolutely Essential Guide to Great BDSM and S&M Sex
*The Absolutely Essential Dominant/submissive Playtime Experience
*The Absolutely Essential BDSM Sexual Experience
*The Ultimate Collection of S&M and BDSM Rules For Female Submissives and Slaves
*Master and submissive or slave BDSM Contract
*The Funniest BDSM Personal Ads
*Have Awesome BDSM Sex
*BDSM Master/slave Contract
*Spanking Dictionary
*BDSM Rules
*Bed Arrest, the Punishment for BDSM Enthusiasts

Book #1

Regularly Spanked, Strapped and Paddled: The Life of a Female Spanking Model

J. Myers

Chapter One

I am spanked professionally. Over the years I developed the ability to take amazingly long, hard spankings.

My father spanked me until I was 18. I was always able to take a hard spanking. When he stopped spanking me I knew I would need to find someone that would. For some reason I respect authority more if they spank me, and that includes my boyfriends and now my masters.

My butt doesn't bruise easily and I take pride in the number of paddles that have been broken over it. Perhaps my ass just doesn't have as many nerve endings as most folk's butts do.

I remember spitefully holding back my tears when being spanked as a child. I look back on that now and realize it was a mistake. I should have faked pain instead of having to deal with the alternative punishments they started giving me.

When I became an adult by chance I gravitated into the BDSM lifestyle as a masochist submissive. Well long story short. I lost my job in the city I lived in, followed my master to this city but later found myself alone and broke. One night while sulking on the bed with only 2 weeks paid on the rent and $45 to my name, I hit on the idea to offer my services as a professional spankee.

I had seen so many professional spankee models' pictures in magazines and on the internet. Many were semi or completely naked while being spanked on video or while being photographed.

I would find clients that wanted to spank me for money, perhaps to help them with their own curiosity, pent-up frustration, anger management, their desire to punish a female, need for stress relief, to relieve addictions, their need for moral forgiveness and/or just for sexual stimulation. I had heard of spanking models offering private play sessions where they were spanked for a fee.

As long as sex is not provided then hopefully it would be legal and not prostitution.

As I told you I was into BDSM and had established contacts here. I had been to play parties and had wowed others with my ability to be spanked. Fortunately I had made friends with a particularly popular master there. I got a hold of his phone number and gave him a call. That call would change my life. I start now from that next day.

I explained to Master Steve what I wanted to do and he said he could help for sure but first wanted me to play with him as a slave. I was not surprised, I was pretty, had a nice body and I knew he wanted to see what I could take. Frankly I needed a good hard play session anyway so I drove over to his house later that day.

Master Steve was himself quite good looking. "Come kneel in front of me young lady" he said glad to see me. I walked over to him with my eyes down. He was sitting on a couch. "Kneel". I knelt in front of him and close to him with my hands behind my head. He removed my top and bra and caressed and played with my tits. "Up higher on your knees young lady" he ordered. My breasts were now at his mouth level and he began sucking away on them. I was already so horny. He pulled both nipples into his mouth and sucked on them. My knees buckled from the pleasure. I don't think it was an orgasm but I continued begging for permission to cum, no such luck.

Master Steve then released my tits and pulled me towards him by the back of my head to kiss him. He stood up and removed his clothing. He then leaned back on the couch, spread his legs and ordered me to suck on his cock.

I had been taught that when I am eating someone or sucking on a cock, I am to stick my butt up and out so it can be enjoyed and otherwise used by others behind me. Also with it up and out, using long implements my ass can be beaten by the person I'm pleasuring. I hadn't seen it when I had originally come over but next to him, Master Steve had already put his long red flogger. I leaned over to Master' cock and sucked on it. I really could suck on cock well, and for a long time. "Harder slave" I heard him say as he rested the flogger on my back. I lapped down Master' ooze, as I licked and sucked. This Master really took care of himself. He ate well, worked out, didn't smoke, etc and I could tell by how good his ooze tasted. I love good tasting ooze and I drank it down eagerly. Suddenly he began flogging my upturned butt as I sucked. FLOP, FLACK...SMACK, CRACK...CRACK, BAM...FLOP, SMACK. The flogger kept landing mostly on my butt but also he flogged my back. He wasn't beating me particularly hard, besides I didn't care because I loved sucking on his cock and the beating was just getting me hornier.

Suddenly it stopped. "Head up young lady." I forced myself to stop sucking and took my head away from his wonderful cock. I kept my eyes on it hoping that being away from it would be just a temporary thing but it was not to be. "I need to see how well your tits deal with being whipped. I've seen you get spanked before but I'll also need to test how well your ass takes a beating too. "Yes Sir." "We'll start with the spanking and then I'll give you the tit whipping. I'm going to love to whip those gorgeous tits of yours." "Yes Master." "Give me your hands." I clapped my hands together on his lap and he tied them securely together. He motioned me to lay over his lap which I did. He began rubbing my butt. "Legs spread". I spread my legs about 2 feet wide. He then stuck his finger up my pussy. Wow did it ever easily slide in. "Wow, you are one wet slave girl. Very good. But no you're not cumming yet."

Master started my spanking with his hand. He went right to work too, *SMACK, BAM, slap, slap, BAM, slap.* I lost count as to how many spanks. Now he was spanking hard, smiling down on me as I squirmed, moaned and cried out. BAM, SPANK, SPANK, BAM, CRACK. I kicked my legs a bit. He was really laying it on fast and furious. Then suddenly I found myself on the verge of cumming. I knew Master wouldn't let me cum so why ask. I continued to yelp, moan and squirm. Suddenly I started cumming even though I didn't mean to. I tried hard not to move my pelvis in a manner that would give away that I was cumming without permission but suddenly Master' hard spanks meant a lot less. Then Master Steve stopped using his hand, reached for a strap and continued the deluge on my ass, rubbing it periodically to admire his work. I had a nice controlled orgasm as he spanked me. *SMACK, BAM...BAM, slap, slap, BAM, SMACK, slap.* I turned back to look at my ass and it was red. "Eyes forward" Master scowled giving me 5 really hard strokes to punctuate it. The spanking now was really hurting and as I had lost concentration, I also lost my orgasm, now all I felt was a lot of pain. *"Ow, noo Master, stop, oow, ow."* I pounded the couch in pain. He was really spanking hard. "Hold your ass still slave." I hadn't realized it but I had lifted my butt up some to avoid the spanks. Wow, that was a bad idea. Master went back to beating my ass and upper legs, this time with a medium size rubber paddle. "Ow, ooh, ooh, pleassee sir, I'llll be good." Dozens of spanks later I was crying. I can take a really hard spanking but all this attention to my posterior was really getting to me. Then suddenly it stopped.

"Kneel" was the order and I eagerly knelt in front of him as I rubbed my butt cheeks. Master bent over me and rubbed my hot butt cheeks. "This is a good test of what you can take." "Yes sir" I moaned. "Now it's time to give those lovely tits of yours the same kind of attention." Oh great, but at least my butt would get a rest for a change.

I had been trained to easily cum from breast stimulation. I am so proud of my breasts. They have given me and others so much pleasure. They can take quite a beating too. Master Steve specialized in tit torture so I suspect my tits would be red soon.

As I knelt in front of him, Master Steve untied my wrists and ordered me to turn around and put my wrists behind my back. He tied my hands behind my back and then ordered me to face him again. He then tied my boobs fairly tightly together at their base. My tits were even firmer than usual now. Their nipples quickly hardened. Master pinched both nipples hard waking me from my dreamy state and making me cry out.

Master then took out a short tit flogger and proceeded to lightly whip my tits with it as I continued to kneel in front of him. I closed my eyes instinctively but the flogger never came anywhere close to my face. Master Steve really knew how to whip tits. Master started to swing from a further distance away thus increasing the velocity. I could tell this was something he really enjoyed doing. This flogging went on for about 5 minutes. Master then put the flogger down and ordered me to turn around, my back now facing him, He now took up the same slapper he had earlier used on my butt. He pulled my head back by the hair exposing my breasts more and proceeded to spank them for real. *Slap, slap,*

slap, slap, slap, slap, slap. Master concentrated spanking the fleshing mounds of the left breast, reaching out, grabbing it by the nipple and separating it from the right breast so more off my large breast was free to spank. It did sting but also felt sinfully good. *Smack...slap, slap, slap, BAM, slap.* Master pinched my left nipple as he held it making me wince but then he twisted it in-between his fingers giving me pleasure. He probably didn't even realize he was playing with the nipple in such a pleasurable way. Giving breasts pleasure and pain is just his nature. I sure wasn't going to complain. Then he let go of my left nipple and got a hold of the right nipple, pulling the right breast out to the right, separating it from its twin, allowing more of it to be beaten. Slap, slap, slap, slap, slap. Blow after blow continued to rain down on my breasts, making them pink and tender. Master pulled up my right breast by the nipple and concentrated his beating on the underside. It did hurt but frankly I was getting more pleasure from a tit whipping from him than when he spanked my ass. I glanced down at my breasts and they were getting red. Suddenly I blurted it out "Master please may I cum?"The whipping stopped suddenly as Master looked at me somewhat puzzled. "Wow, I love how masochistic you are." He them grabbed both of my large nipples together with one hand and pulled my breasts up exposing their soft underbelly, going to work on them both at once with the slapper and spanking them hard now. *"Ow, ohh no Master, ow, oww, oh pleeaaseee Master."* Slap...slap, slap...slap, slap. He let go of my tits. He then proceeded to spank their upper front. "Folks are going to love whipping your tits" "Yes Master." This was hurting now and I wasn't going to be allowed to cum so I was going to just have to take it.

My breasts were now a shade of red and Master Steve stopped. I thought my tit whipping was over but I was wrong. "Turn around slave." I turned around obediently and knelt there as he untied my wrists. Then in my stupor I remembered that there was another position for me and my tits to be whipped in...and more.

Master, himself now naked, lead me over to the half table and ordered me to climb on it and lay on my back. The half table is many feet long with long vertical brackets so my legs are kept in place securely. My arms and waist are strapped down to the table.

My d-cup breasts thus are fully exposed and securely in place should they be the focus of attention, as they often are. On the half table my pussy and asshole are right on the edge of the table so they can be played with and taken with ease. My former master put me in one of these half tables at a friend's house often and left me there for his and sometimes other's pleasure. With my legs in this position I can easily be spanked and taken both in my pussy and ass.

Master tied each leg to the table's built-in leg braces. A strap came over my waist to keep it in place and straps held each wrist and upper arm in place. I was now quite vulnerable and immobile. I was also blindfolded. But for the time being Master Steve was a lot more interested in finishing the job he started with my breasts. Now though he would use the big black flogger to beat them.

Master bent down to my pussy and sucked the copious amount of cum out of it. "You know what's coming now young lady don't you." "Yes sir" I think I said. He raised the flogger and CRACK. "Ow". CRACK, CRACK...SMACK. This is a big room so Master could raise up the big flogger and let it fly. CRACK, CRACK...SMACK, BAM...SMACK, BAM. I was trying to move away but to no avail. I was held too tightly in place and could go nowhere. BAM, SMACK, BAM. Master was working up a sweat and loving every second of it. I was so exposed and I knew by now my pussy was dripping wet. I couldn't wait for him to take me. Hopefully he'll take me for a long time too. I held onto that thought as the blows rained down on my chest. *"Master, please, ohh, ahhh."* Master was very skilled and the flogger never landed more than a couple of inches above my breasts. Finally it was over.

He now played with my sensitive breasts grabbing, kneading, twisting, turning and holding them. "I am so proud of my work and your breasts are so much fun to work with. People are going to pay good money to beat you." Well I guess that's good. I had bills. "Thank you sir." I muttered. Master bent down and lightly bite my nipples one by one, also sucking on them and playing with my breasts more. He clearly loved my tits. Suddenly I remembered what could come next, yes, it could be the highlight of my day.

I looked down at my chest and it was a red. My nipples were hot and sensitive. I heard Master doing something and I looked over at him. He had made himself hard and was coming over to my exposed holes. First he got out some Vaseline and used his finger to lubricate my anus. He inserted his finger deep into it making me moan in anticipation. He then cleaned off his finger with alcohol and a paper towel. "Beg for it slave" he ordered. "Master please take me." "You can do better than that." "Master I'm begging, please take me and fuck me hard." Then he entered my pussy. Immediately I began begging to cum, which he allowed me to do.

Master grabbed my upper legs to hold me in place while he pounded my pussy. I came so hard. I lost track of what time it was. "Come harder slut" he roared and I did just that pumping my hips against him as he took me. I couldn't wait for him to take me in my ass. "You like how this feels in that naughty little cunt of yours don't you slave." "Yes sir" I stammered. He pounded me harder and buried the strap-on in my pussy, just leaving it there for a few moments as he gyrated his hips, making his cock move from side to side. I was so wet that it slide easily in my pussy. "Wow, you're one soaking wet little slave girl." I couldn't answer though I think I tried. I was cumming so hard. About then he pulled out of my pussy and stuck the strap-on in my ass. *"Ohhhhh Master, yes, thank you....ohhh."* He started taking me slowly in the ass at first but built up speed and after a couple of minutes was pounding my butthole with vigor. I felt no pain, just waves of ecstasy.

Master finished taking me a while later and cleaned off his equipment as I lay tied down exhausted and helpless. He left me there with my spread legs up in the air. My tits a shade of red and my ass somewhat sore and tender. He went to the couch and we talked about my being a professional spankee.

Master Steve was impressed by how much abuse my body could take and was confident I could make a decent living doing this. I didn't bruise that much which would be helpful. It was important though that I don't have sex if I took money. Amazingly he actually thought that as long as sexual favors were not offered, the law was more on my side if a client tried to abuse me. Of course if the police were called I would now be in their sights which would not be to my benefit.

For the next hour he kept me tied to the half table checking to see how my body dealt with the beatings. He also took the opportunity to take me again before releasing me. In exchange for regularly being his sex slave, he promised to help me and even said he could get me 2 clients immediately. He even said he'd spread the word that I was a friend of his cousin, a city policeman.

Advice he gave was:

*Don't sexually play with them or let them take liberties sexually with my body
*If they want to masturbate after spanking me, let them but I shouldn't ever masturbate around a client.
*Use an online phone number that would be difficult to trace
*Get the cash up front
*Don't use my real name.
*Spankings could only be done using their hands, unless they pay extra
*Ideally they need to be recommended to me by someone I trust.
*Give my butt and/or tits enough time to heal in between clients.
*If I breakdown and have sex with a client, even touch them sexually, or vice versa, I have to give them their money back
*Have a safe word and make sure they understand my limits
*Tit whipping would cost extra.

Master Steve released me and we had something to eat on his porch. That would be the last time he would beat me for some time. When I came over to be his sex toy though he loved seeing all the marks on my body and where it was red. He would be a comforting friend and lover during this busy period of my life.

Three days later I had a bruise-free ass and my first gig.

Chapter Two

Master got me my first client, Rick. I knew him from a play party. I also knew he was a veteran spanker thus knew how to spank. We agreed on the terms and a time that night and the price of $100. I drove over to his place.

Unexpectedly Rick had a friend there, John. John had never spanked a girl before and was interested in it. As agreed I took the cash as I walked in and sat on the couch in his living room waiting for the inevitable spanking.

We first all had some wine. He then brought a wooden spanking horse out for me to bend over. It had straps for the spankee but Master Steve had previously made it plain that I don't allow myself to be strapped in, unless he was there. I would first get spanked OTK by both of them and then get spanked over the wooden spanking horse.

The truth was that I didn't know what the definition of a full, complete spanking was and they wondered themselves. I told them that my butt can be red.

I was told to lay over Rick's lap, which I did. Rick raised my skirt and pulled my panties down and off. He massaged and kneaded my ass for some time as he talked to John. Wow, that massaging felt good but for both of our sakes I had to do all I could to keep this legal so I kept my legs closed. Then he started spanking. *Slap, slap, slap, BAM, slap, crack, slap, bam, slap, Bam.* This was a basic warm-up spanking which I was grateful for. Rick explained the importance of a warm up spanking to John but he added *when a girl was going to get spanked for some time.* Apparently he wanted to get his hundred dollar's worth. I gulped but I guess that's what they're supposed to be able to do to a professional spankee.

Spank, spank, slap, spank, slap, BAM, slap, crack, SMACK. I squirmed a bit and repositioned myself for a long stay over his lap. He spanked with a steady rhythm. *Spank, smack, smack, slap, smack.* I began softly moaning after the 20th spank and the noises I would make grew progressively louder from then on. He concentrated on the right cheek for some time, then the left cheek but my butt could outlast a lot of spankers and soon he was shifting from his tired right hand to left hand and then back to his right hand. *"Owww, ohh, ahhh."* Still the spanking went on and on and hurt! *SMACK, bam, bam, slap, slap, SMACK.* Then he stopped and I caught my breath. I hadn't started crying but was getting quite a charge from the spanking. He on the other hand was tired. How great was that. I still laid there over his lap and actually he continued to hold me firmly in place. Sure enough round 2 was about to begin.

Rick called John over who brought a chair and sat across from him. I was now in-between them, lucky me. John then started spanking the cheek closest to him and Rick spanked the cheek closest to him. *Spank, SMACK, spank, SPANK, spank, spank, spank, crack, SMACK.* Should I be charging more for this duo spanking stuff?

"It's amazing how tough your butt is, all there is is some redness" said John, impressed. *Slap, spank, BAM, slap, crack, spank, bam.* John spanked down my upper leg and Rick told him to stay on my butt. *Spank, crack, spank, bam.* It was hurting significantly now *"Ahhh, ohhh, owww"* I said. The spanks landed 2-3 a second with both of them spanking me. *Spank, spank, spank, bam, slap, Bam.* I began kicking my feet up and down a foot or two, much to their delight. I know I also was giving them a great view of my anus and pussy as modesty was no longer a priority as my butt reddened.

My spanking had lasted about 30 minutes and I looked back and saw that my butt was red. I was crying out with every spank now. A good spanking leaves the spankee with a red butt so I worked up the courage to say okay guys that that was enough. A minute or so later the spanking stopped.

I wanted to get up but Rick wanted to use his fingernails to rake my hot, red butt before massaging it for a while. I never thought of that but I would have to get used to that after the spanking stops. The raking of the butt didn't hurt as much as the actual spanking of course and after all admiring their work would be exciting for them and less painful for me than the actual spanking. I submissively kept on lying across his lap. Both massaged my butt and wow did it feel good but I knew where somebody's hand was going to go. "Please guys, only my butt, it stays legal that way." Well I hoped that was how it stayed legal anyway. John got to rake and massage the cheek he worked his magic on and Rick got to rake and massage the cheek he spent the most time on.

I put my hands back on the carpet and waited for them to be through. I guess for $100 they deserve to relax that way.

We made some small talk and John got my wine and brought it to me as I continued to lay over Rick's lap. I asked Rick if I could get up and he said no. Well it was $100 he spent so I laid there. Finally he had to go to the bathroom and my first spanking for money was over.

Fortunately I loved the feeling of a sensitive, sore well-spanked butt rubbing against my panties. Good thing because I would have a sore butt quite a bit from now on. I was grateful that my first spanking gig went well. Rick knew Master Steve and wanted to stay in good graces with this town's BDSM community. He was also a good guy. I could only hope I would be so lucky from now on with my clients.

A problem however could be that spankings does turn me on but I knew that I had to give them back the money if I had sex with them and I had promised myself sexually to Master Steve.

Word of mouth is such a powerful business force. I had left cards with the guys and got a call from someone they knew 3 days later.

His name was Brad and was a business associate of Master Steve's. He actually was in town for only a short time. We chatted on specifics and set a time for me to come over that night. Once again I would get a good, long spanking.

I met Brad at the hotel bar and we chatted. I was a good listener and I would find that was a real asset in this line of work. After a while we went up to his room. I went in to use the bathroom and came out and he was naked. I wanted to ask him to put his cloths back on but just gave up. He already knew he couldn't play with me. He sat on the bed and I, still fully clothed, I laid over his lap.

No matter how many spankings I have gotten in life I still get butterflies in my stomach when I'm about to get another good one. I was now in my familiar position of lying over a man's lap, butt up, with my hands on the floor and feet hanging down the other end. The dress I had worn was a short, thin, sexy one. It's important to keep the client hungry for you as $100 is a good deal of money. He massaged my fully clothed butt and upper legs, apparently in no hurry to start the spanking. Then he pulled up my dress, massaging my panty-covered butt for a bit and then pulled my panties all the way off of me. Brad explained to me that he hadn't had sex in months since he separated from his girlfriend. Once again I explained how for everybody's legal protection I couldn't have sex or engage in sexual activities. That usually stops them. Unfortunately keeping them from trying to have sex with me would be a regular part of the job and frankly got old.

Brad spanking started with more intensity than I expected. *Spank, spank, spank, slap, slap, crack.* My butt was no longer sore from the spanking several days ago so it needed a bit of breaking in again. Slap, crack, spank, spank, spank."*Ohhhhhh*" I muttered unexpectedly as the spanking continued. He ordered me to give him my right hand and he held it firmly to my lower back making it tougher for me to move around. "Young lady I'm going to turn this lovely ass a very nice shade of red." *Spank, spank, spank, slap, bam.* "Oww, ohhhh." My feet started kicking as he picked up the pace of the spanking. Instinctively I squeezed my butt cheeks together and tightened them up. He seemed to spank harder when I did that though. *"Ahh, ohh."* "Do you think I'm capable of giving you a good spanking young lady" he asked clearly enjoying beating my ass. "Yes sir" I said in-between spanks. Wow, he could spank, he wasn't missing a beat, though he was switching off to his other hand periodically. *Spank, slap, slap, bam, BAM.* "Now we're getting somewhere. You're butts getting red, but it's got a ways to go."

You just never know what the guy's going to become like when he's spanking. He was quite the gentleman down at the bar when we first met but now was a tiger, still I was getting spanked so what did I expect. *"Ow, ow, oh....oh...ow."* Well I had officially entered the serious pain zone. I looked back at my ass and he was right, it was getting red. I also realized I had become horny and now that I was kicking my feet with a bit more gusto, he could easily see my anus and pussy. I tried to close my legs but the spanking was too intense. He unexpectedly stopped spanking but he wasn't letting me up. I quickly tried to get up but was held down. 'No young lady, this spanking is not over. You lay still" he said very firmly. I wanted to say that that was enough of a spanking but he was so firm with me that I was scared to. I waited for the inevitable to continue. He rubbed my red ass all the way down my legs. His hands almost brushed my pussy. It felt good but I knew I had to stay on guard. He raked my sore ass with his fingernails then the kneading and massaging of my well spanked ass continued. It was a very nice break but the problem was his spanking muscles were getting recharged for round 2, and then along came round two and now he was really spanking hard. *SPANK, SPANK, Spank, spank, spank, slap, BAM.* I kicked my legs as my now sensitive red cheeks bounced up and down from the blows. I pushed up on his leg with my free hand as I tried feebly to get away but he held me too tight. The blows rained down on my exposed ass. I cried out with each blow. He was really going for it. *"Ow, owwwww...ohhh...oww."* SPANK SPANK, SPANK, spank, spank, BAM, BAM. Then suddenly he stopped. He was breathing hard and my ass really hurt.

He just looked down at me, massaging my hot, red ass. Then he raked both cheeks again with his dull but significant sized fingernails. That caught me off guard. I caught my breath. I felt the cool air in the hotel room on my ass. I wasn't sure who was going to speak first. Finally I spoke. "That was really quite a spanking." I suddenly realized though that he had a very tight grip on me and I wasn't going to be able to get up unless he let go of me. "I'm going to have to get up now" I said. As if in a trance he suddenly came to and released me. I slipped off his lap and came to rest on my knees on the carpet below him, immediately rubbing my sore butt vigorously. I would have been a nice sight as he looked down at me. I was instinctively looking at his cock, I really wanted to suck on it but I knew the law and really needed the money. He just sat there looking down at me. His cock was hard and staring at me. I pushed myself up using his knees all the while looking at it. I bent down and got my panties and put them on.

This no sex rule was going to be tough for me to enforce but I knew it was the right thing to do.

I gingerly sat down across from him on one of the room's double beds and we talked. He was actually a neat guy to talk to. I congratulated him on really getting his money's worth as I fidgeted while sitting. He tried to seduce me, even offering me more money but I said grudgingly that I was really sorry but couldn't. Soon I left that much closer to paying rent.

That next day I called Master Steve to thank you him for the contact and ask him when he next wanted me to come over and serve him. Happily he said in an hour and gave me instructions on what to wear and what to do.

I got there in the skirt and blouse he ordered me to wear. I wasn't allowed to wear underwear but thankfully could wear a bra as the blouse he wanted me to wear was somewhat see-through. I let myself in as instructed and immediately went and kneeled in front of him. We talked for a while as he undressed me. He then had me lay over his lap so he could inspect my ass. It was still marked and a little red from last night's spanking. It was firmer too. My butt gets firm from being well spanked. He was really impressed and would later call Brad and congratulate him on a job well done. He massaged my ass and teased my pussy for a bit with a vibrator but sadly wouldn't let me cum.

Master would have loved to have tied me up naked and beaten me, and frankly other than on the butt, I wouldn't have minded either but I had to be as mark-free as possible. He did however still have a lot he could do with my body. I was ordered to put my hands behind the small of my back and he tied them together. I then was ordered to sit in front of him so his chest was against my back. He then commenced playing with my breasts. It felt so good. I started to say something but he ordered me to be silent. He then took out a bottle of massage oil, put big globs on both his hands and commenced to massage my breasts using the lubrication of the massage oil. Within 20 seconds I was ready to cum. I asked for permission and got it. *"Ahhhhh, yes, ohhhhhhhhh."* As my hands were tied behind my back, and I was up against Master, I was able to play with his cock and instinctively I did. He wasn't real hard but soon would be. Using his hands, Master Steve ran circles around the lubricated fleshy part of my breasts for many minutes making me beg to have my nipples played with. *"Master Steve please play with my nipples so I can cum harder for you."* That was the way to ask a Master as he suddenly did and my body shook from the intenseness of the orgasm. *"Awwwwwww yessssss, awwwwww."* Waves of pleasure rolled over me and I strained at my bonds as the spasms engulfed me. *"Awwwwww."* 20 minutes of this came and went and like all good things, it ended. But what a divine interlude it was.

Then he then ordered me to turn around and slide down to his cock and put my mouth to good use.

It's a good thing I have such a strong mouth as Master had me sucking for a long time. He came and I remained there with his cock in my mouth for around 10 minutes to make sure to drink up all of his cum.

After that he took me to his bedroom and I massaged him for around an hour. He then decided he would take me after-all.

I was ordered to go to the half-table, the table I was strapped down to and taken last time I was here. Thank goodness. I really wanted him to take me.

As previously noted, the half table is many feet long with stirrups so my legs are kept in place securely. My arms and waist are strapped down to the table. My breasts are fully exposed and securely in place. On the half table my pussy and asshole are right on the edge of the table so they can be played with and taken with ease. With my legs in this position I can easily be taken both in my pussy and ass.

Master tied each leg to the table's built-in stirrups. A strap came over my waist to keep it in place and straps held each wrist and upper arm in place. I was now quite vulnerable and immobile. I was also blindfolded.

Master bent down to my pussy and sucked the copious amount of cum out of it. I begged to be allowed to cum and he let me. He pulled over a chair and kept eating me as he decided what he wanted to do next with me. I and my still warm pink bottom were completely at his disposal. I came hard. I thought maybe Master would whip my tits like he really enjoys doing but he was kind enough to spare them in case they were to get whipped while I work. He stopped eating me and I knew what would happen next. It would be the highlight of my day.

I heard Master doing something and I looked over at him. He had gotten hard and was coming over to my exposed holes. First he got out some Vaseline and used his finger to lubricate my anus. He inserted his finger deep into it making me moan in anticipation. He then cleaned off his finger with a paper towel and rubbing alcohol. "Beg for it slave" he ordered. "Master please take me with your big hard cock". "You can do better than that." "Master I'm begging, please take me with your big hard cock and fuck me hard because I need to be fucked hard by Master to clear my head." Then he entered my pussy. Immediately I began begging to cum, which he allowed me to do.

Master grabbed my upper legs to hold me in place while he pounded my pussy with his cock. I came so hard. "Come harder slut" he roared and I did just that pumping my hips against him as he took me. I couldn't wait for him to take me in my ass. "You like how this feels in that naughty little cunt of yours don't you slave." "Yes sir" I stammered. He pounded me harder and buried his cock in my pussy, just leaving it there for a few moments as he gyrated his hips, making it move from side to side. I was so wet that it easily slide in my pussy. "Wow, you're one soaking wet little slave girl." I couldn't answer, though I think I tried. I was cumming so hard. A few minutes after he pulled out of my pussy and stuck his cock in my ass. *"Ohhhhh Master, yes, thank you....ohhh."* He started taking me slowly in the ass at first but built up speed and after a couple of minutes was pounding my butthole with vigor. I felt no pain, just waves of ecstasy.

Master finished taking me a while later and left me tied down exhausted and helpless. He left me there with my spread legs up in the air and went about his business. I dozed off.

Chapter Three

I got a call from Master a few days later. He had a couple of guys that wanted to spank me and would pay $300 but insisted on using implements. He said I would be spanked really hard. They would do it at his place. I would spend a lot of the spanking tied up naked to the half table. I was reluctant to say no to any of his requests and after being assured that there wouldn't be any sex, I agreed. It would happen that night and I should be wearing a schoolgirl outfit when I got there.

I knew this would be a real hard spanking that would make me cry hard. It made me scared and I had butterflies in my stomach for the rest of the day. It was as if I knew I was going to be punished later by a parent or master and really wished it could be over with already. My marks from the previous spanking had gone so at least they would start with a fresh ass, something no doubt they'd like. The truth is that I loved being strapped down to the half table and at least Master would be there to watch things. Hopefully he could keep his hands off me sexually too, at least until after the two guys were gone.

I got there in my schoolgirl outfit looking very cute. I had put my hair in pigtails, something I hadn't done in a while. The guys were there and I nervously looked at them. Sadly they looked pretty strong, but at least they were good looking.

I sat down on a chair between Tim and Frank. Master brought me a glass of wine. We chatted. They seemed pretty nice but I know how guys can get when they start spanking, they become animals. They wanted to see my butt so I took off my skimpy panties and backed to one, then the other, lifting up my schoolgirl skirt when I got to each. They enjoyed feeling it, massaging it, kneading it and I stayed in front of each until they told me they were done. I told them that I had had butterflies in my stomach all day anticipating this.

"Your ass is a perfect ass for spanking" one said. Oh lucky me.

I'd been there for about 30 minutes and Master came over and sat on the couch. Sternly he ordered me to strip, which I did. My nipples were already erect knowing what was to come.

I stood before them naked. I then was ordered to go over to Master who tied my hands together in front of me. I then told the guys that I expected to cry from this and that it was okay.

What was to come was one of the longest and hardest spankings I've ever had.

I was instructed to lie over Frank's lap which I did. Frank didn't waste any time and got right into spanking me. Oh did I forget to mention that he had big hands? *SPANK, spank, bam, bam, spank, slap, spank.* I hunkered down to be soundly beaten. *Bam, bam, spank, slap.* I tried not to raise my feet this early in the spanking and kept thinking about the $300 I would make from this. Rent and utilities would be paid for this month and just in the nick of time too. Then frank gave me 5 of his hardest and it made me yell out. "Ahhhhhhh." They all had a laugh. "Ow that hurt" I said more for the fun of it than anything. Frank rubbed my butt again for a bit and got back to the spanking. *Slap, SMACK, slap, SMACK, slap, BAM, slap, crack, SMACK. "Ohhhh……ahhhh".* He was spanking harder now and really enjoying himself. I sucked in air and clenched my fingers as serious pain had officially kicked in. If only I could cum from it. I needed to try and cum. It would make the spanking a lot more enjoyable. I tried rubbing his leg inconspicuously then he hit me with those 5 super hard ones again. BAM, BAM, BAM, BAM, BAM. *"Ahhhhh, owwww."* I was now always crying out from the spanking. Then it stopped. Frank rubbed my butt, also grabbing handfuls of butt cheek which hurt actually. He was pleased with his work but fair is fair and it was Tim's turn for me to lay over his lap and be spanked. I was ordered to get up and lay over Tim's lap. Oh that felt great, not only had the spanking stopped for precious seconds but I got to move my butt, but with my hands tied in front of me I couldn't rub it. I slowly walked over to Tim who ordered me to "hurry up". I laid over his lap and, well here we go again.

Tim spanked in a hold different way. I don't think he had done much if any spanking before. The good news is that he wasn't spanking hard. He spanked all over my butt, top left cheek, then next spank was bottom right cheek, then the middle of a cheek, etc. It was kind of neat actually. "So what does my butt look like?" I asked for the fun of it now that I wasn't crying out in pain from every spank. "A little pink; it's a nice start anyway" Tim said reminding me that the festivities of the night were just starting and my butt was the main event. Spank, spank, spank, slap, BAM, slap, crack, SMACK. *"Owww."* I scrunched my toes and now made regular yelps as he really was spanking hard now.

Before I knew it around 10 minutes had passed and I was crying. I was then ordered to get up off of Tim's lap. I so wanted to rub my now bruised well spanked butt and didn't care that I was naked and everybody was gazing at my full frontal nudity. Of course I couldn't as I my hands were tied in front of me. "Does it hurt yet young lady?" Frank asked sarcastically. "Yes" I quickly answered. They smiled. Then the guys started walking towards the half table. Master was already there. "Get on the table young lady" Master said and I grudgingly started walking over there. As I walked by Frank though he put his arm out across my stomach so I was kept checked in place while he ran his other hand over my ass. "Nice warm ass". He let me go and I walked over the half table and climbed on and lay on my back. My legs were put in the stirrups and held securely in place with straps. My hands were untied and then my arms and waist were strapped down to the table. I was also blindfolded. On the half table my ass was right on the edge of the table so it can be beaten with ease. I was now quite vulnerable and immobile. Then much to my surprise, Master brought over a ball gag and gagged me. I knew Master had a sadistic streak in him and it then dawned on me how he was really going to enjoy seeing me get beaten like this. I hadn't counted on being gagged but too late now.

I don't know who was doing it but both ass cheeks were getting raked, rubbed, pinched and kneaded. The problem was that some bumping of my pussy lips and anus was occurring whether it was intentional or not and I showed my concern by making a lot of noise through my gag and moving around as much as I could being so well strapped down to the table. They got the hint and their hands stayed from then on my ass.

Then suddenly it stopped. I had been so concerned about where their hands were that I forgot what was in store for me. Oh god, here it comes. CRACK. Oh no, both had a strap and were staggering their swats. One gave me a spank from one side and the other gave me a swat from the other side. The first blow landed smack down the middle of both cheeks. It was a wonderfully aimed spank I must admit but hurt so much. I lurched all I could being strapped down so tight. My constant yells were muffled by the gag. The strapping though continued and it hurt something fierce. CRACK, CRACK, CRACK, CRACK, BAM, BAM. My ass and now upper legs were being beaten by the straps, and non-stop. The sound the strap made when it landed on my ass reverberated through the room. CRACK, CRACK, CRACK. It could be my worst beating in months. SMACK, BAM, BAM...SMACK, SMACK, BAM. I bet all my muffled crying was making their cocks hard. Someone grabbed my legs and lifted my ass higher exposing more ass to spank. The strapping continued. SMACK, SMACK, SMACK, BAM, BAM, BAM, BAM. I tried to move my ass but it was too securely in place. My ass was pulled out and up as far as the pelvic strap would allow all in an effort to expose as much ass as possible. SMACK, SMACK, SMACK, BAM, BAM. Frank and Tim were in heaven, they could now really beat a slave girl like they had always dreamed of. I could not escape the blows that were raining down on my ass. Tears were running down my cheeks. I can usually take a good beating but as sensitive as my ass was already and with such a beating on my tender ass with straps, was too much. I know this spanking will leave so many marks on my ass and I didn't expect to be able to sit.

The spanking stopped. I so hoped it had ended. My ass still was on fire. I felt cold hands massaging it as I kept crying from the lingering pain. I pulled on my wrist straps. I was ready for this to end but the blindfold and gag held. What I didn't know is that the two guys had exchanged their straps for paddles and the deluge on my ass would now once again begin. *SMACK, CRACK, SPANK, SPANK, SPANK*. I was already crying so I now just cried harder. I clenched my butt cheeks but doing just that really hurt and then there were the blows raining down on my clenched cheeks. I thought about trying to cum from the pain but it hurt too much. Also it was now difficult to think of anything but the pain. Oh god if there was something they wanted me to stop doing I promise I will. I'll be such a good girl. SPANK, SPANK...SMACK, SPANK, SPANK. I heard them talking but I couldn't make out what they said. They were stopping now more often and rubbing my butt in-between swats and occasionally adjusting my blindfold to make sure it covered my eyes completely. After around 15 minutes more of off and on paddling, it stopped. I remained strapped down helpless. I also remained crying. After more massaging of my butt the voices became more distant. Was it over yet? I also became aware of wetness running down my ass crack. I had become so wet that that it was running down from my pussy. No doubt that was an exciting sight for everybody.

Then they came back and this time each took a turn individually with the paddle. I couldn't believe it. I just kept crying. What else could I do? I'm so glad the ball gag was on me because all my crying had become embarrassing. In time the spanking ended but my crying continued. My ass was so sore.

I remained strapped down to the half table. Soon though I didn't hear the guy's voices and I knew the spanking had ended. I tried hard and was able to stop crying finally. I remained strapped down to the half table whimpering on and off. I was exhausted. I figured Master would let me up soon which was a saving grace. I think I even fell asleep.

I was awoken by a mouth sucking on my pussy, drinking up my cum. I had to assume it was Master. The ball gag was still on me as well as the blindfold. My ears were actually ringing. I didn't know why. Then the pussy eating got really intense. I hoped it was master because I had no strength to resist. Magically a vibrator appeared and I came so hard. I forgot about my intense beating and so incredibly sore ass and shook with such an intense orgasm. Master ran the vibrator along my clit then entered me while massaging me with the vibrator. Oh man was that ever intense. I don't know where I found the energy but I had such an uncontrollable orgasm. The truth is that I don't know when it ended because I passed out or fell asleep at some point.

When I woke up I noticed that I could see light. Not only was the blindfold was off me but I was also unstrapped, good thing because I had to go to the bathroom quick. I ran in and sat on the toilet and *owwwwww*. I forgot about my severely spanked ass. I would need to take care when sitting for a while. I climbed into bed with Master and that would be it for that wild night's experience.

I slept in the next day and was tired through much of it. Master and I had sex twice as both of us were really horny. Master invited some BDSM friends over to see my butt. It was a work of art and frankly I was very proud of it. He counted 14 bruises and even late that afternoon it was still reddish. People *ewwed and ahhed*. Nobody had ever seen a butt the next day that well spanked. That night Frank even came over to see his handiwork. I was kind of scared to see him actually but he promised it was just to look and not to spank. He too was really impressed and we took pictures that only showed my butt. I would later use those pictures to help get clients.

I went home the next day and continued to give my butt a well deserved rest.

Chapter Four

4 nights later I got a call from someone that nobody knew. As nobody knew him I decided against meeting him. He would call again though.

About a week later most of my bruises were gone and good thing as Master had a new client for me and he would become a regular.

We talked on the phone and I told him how he had to spank with his hand and other specifics. He agreed. Once again I would go to Master' house for it which was my preference anyway. I had come to realize that Master really enjoyed watching others spank me and spank me hard. I guess the arrangement worked to my favor as I was safer there and I could have sex with him legally afterwards, something I really needed after a good spanking.

The truth was I hadn't been spanked in a week and I really needed it. I'm a spankophile and even after that extreme spanking I had, I remained addicted to being spanked. Frankly the lingering pain from that spanking made me horny. I kind of missed it. Obviously being a spankophile comes in handy if one is a professional spankee.

I got in a sexy dress, put on my make-up, got the high heels on and drove over to Master'. I hung out watching TV but Tom never showed up. He called an hour later and apologized and asked to re-schedule for tomorrow. Master added $40 for my wasted time and gasoline tonight and he agreed. Tomorrow came along and he called Master and said he was willing to pay $200 total but wanted to use a small paddle on me instead of his hand. Master agreed to it, not consulting me, but such is life. As I have noted Master loves to see me spanked hard. Imagine my surprise though when I got there that night to find out I was going to get a good paddling, not just a good spanking. Still $200 would be nice to have and I really did want a spanking so here we go again.

Come nightfall I got all the sexy clothing back on and went back to Master' house, not sure he would even show up. He did, though he was 25 minutes late. He put the money on the TV, I took it and put it in my purse.

I really didn't know what to think of him. He wasn't shaved but didn't smell. Master gave him a drink (oh that's another thing about getting spanked at Master's place, he throws in free drinks!) We talked about how I loved to be spanked and his spanking experience with adults and I guess he had plenty. Okay well so what now. He looked over at Master and asked how to proceed. That was nice of him. Master told me to lay over his lap which I did.

Just the thought of being spanked had made me wet and frankly I had been horny all day thinking about it. If he hadn't shown up tonight I would have begged Master for a spanking.

As I lay over his lap he commented about what a beautiful sight I was which was nice. He then slid his hand down and cupped a boob. Oh shit. I jumped off and knelt in front of him, frustrated. I hesitated for a few seconds and then told him that the spanking couldn't happen tonight as it could be considered prostitution. He apologized. Master reluctantly agreed. It was now uncomfortable with him being there. I went and got his money out of my purse and gave it back to him. There was silence in the room and finally he got up and left.

Sure I was frustrated not having the money but what if he was a cop. I also had another problem. I was horny and really wanted a spanking. Master bless his heart was there to lend a helping hand. He ordered me to strip and I eagerly laid over his lap. I had to cum from being spanked he said and I would too. It wasn't a hard spanking at all, in fact fairly light. It didn't leave any marks for sure but it thankfully lasted about 20 minutes. Master let me stay overnight and thankfully later played with me with a vibrator. I of course reciprocated by making good use of my mouth on his cock.

A few days later Jack called for the first time and left a message. Jack is a very nice senior citizen who was looking for an adult school girl to lecture and punish. I would drive to his place in a schoolgirl outfit or something girlish and act like a scared young lady. He would lecture me about something, give me a good spanking, though not too hard, and send me into the corner. Usually I would get 3 spankings in-between my corner time and being lectured. Due to his age perhaps he didn't seem to have a strong sex drive and his groping me would not often be a problem. I sometimes would not charge him and throw in a blow job and/or hand job with the spankings as I know he needed it at least periodically. He would thankfully become a regular and I counted on him to spank me almost as often as I wanted. In fact I often called him up and asked him if he wanted a session with me. Sometimes he'd go to Master' house to watch me get spanked by him (and even join in the fun.)

Regulars like Jack are the thing to have, particularly when they would leave me alone sexually. I started specializing in bad schoolgirl fantasies for older men and always was able to pay my bills.

Well off to my next spanking. See ya!

The End

Book #2 - Bed Arrest, the Punishment for BDSM Enthusiasts

By Phil G.

Copyright (C) 2013

Bed Arrest, the Punishment for BDSM Enthusiasts

Trust, care, mutual consent, safe sex practices, and general safety are absolute priorities. No matter what it's suggested that you incorporate at least the following into your playtime and lifestyle:

* Don't tie things around someone's neck, and no breath play, period!
* Create a "Safe word" for the submissive to say when (or if) things get too scary.
* Always be careful and take necessary safety precautions when engaging in BDSM activity. Keep proper medical facilities handy.
* Always insure that a bound person has adequate circulation. If the person tied up has to go to the bathroom or has physical problems, that person must be immediately released from bondage.
* Ask about medical issues before playing and adjust your playing activities according to any medical issues.
* Never leave anyone bound and alone.
* Understand what a gagged person sounds like in sexual ecstasy versus in pain.
* Do not play while under the influence of drugs or alcohol.
Always check that your handcuffs and/or lock keys work before playing. If you have to go to the locksmith to get the handcuffs off, it's going to be embarrassing.
* When removing someone from bondage, allow them to move their own limbs.
* If pregnant or ill, check with your doctor before engaging in BDSM related activity.
* Always play within your own skill base and comfort level.

Defining Bed Arrest

Thank you for reading this book, the first book on bed arrest.

This punishment technique can only be used when all parties involved have fully consented to it.

For consistency's sake, this book discusses bed arrest where the punisher is a male master and the person being sentenced to bed arrest is a female submissive or slave. Bed arrest as a punishment can however work just as well in situations when the two parties involved are of the same sex.

I am honored to say that as a master I have incorporated bed arrest into my relationships many times. I have found that it can be a useful tool for changing errant sub/slave behavior.

In this book I'll also make suggestions regarding how (in my opinion) to most optimally carry out the sentence of bed arrest on a sub/slave. Obviously both parties involved can adapt what's in this book to fit their desires, needs and time schedule.

This book also assumes (for all involved) that the sub/slave will accept being put in bed arrest and obey her master's rules associated with it. Obviously if master tells his sub/slave she's just been sentenced to 10 hours house arrest and she points at him and laughs, then master has a problem.

General Definition - Bed arrest is when a master in a BDSM (or related) relationship orders (thus requires) his sub/slave to stay on her bed at all times other than emergencies, and for those additional activities specified. During the time that she is reprimanded to the bed, master may also punish her in other ways such as spanking. He can also play with her, and of course enjoy her sexually.

Bed arrest, as is obvious, is a lot like an adult version of timeout. It doesn't need to be for a longtime; a 30 minute bed arrest session might get the point across just as well. Still all bed arrests sessions are not the same and the sub's restrictions during her incarceration can make all the difference in the world. However beware guys, with her helplessly stuck there, will you be able to resist playing with her all afternoon? (Let's hope she doesn't consider that punishment.)

During bed arrest her freedom can be seriously restricted and she will have time to think about the importance of changing her errant ways.

I gave many 2 day sentences as well as 30 minute sentences. The longest bed arrest sentence I ever given a sub/slave was 4 days. On many occasions I commuted the sentence down because of good behavior, and/or something unexpected came up and/or her sexy begging finally got to me.

Bed arrest in and of itself might not be considered that extreme a punishment. The liberties that the sub/slave loses during bed arrest as well as other punishments she might also experience during that time perhaps can better determine how well she learns her lesson.

1. When to use bed arrest as a punishment. Perhaps your lovely lady has not been reacting well enough to your usual punishments. Perhaps spanking her used to work well as a punishment but now she gets so turned on by it that if anything she'll misbehave to get a good spanking. Finding a new punishment thus has become a necessity.

2. Length of time for putting the sub/slave in bed arrest. Obviously this varies by what extent she needs to be punished and what her and her master's obligations in life are during that time. (Does she have to go to work? Does she have college classes, etc.?)

As she will be allowed out of the bed (and home) for work and other responsibilities, likely that would mean an increase in the length of her sentence as she would be spending less time in bed arrest overall than a sub/slave that could stay around the home all or most of the day.

My experience (and yours may be quite different) is that if the sub/slave has never served a bed arrest, she may have fantasies associated with it.

3. What the sub/slave is allowed to do during bed arrest – How strict and restrictive will her sentence be, at least for the first half or so? Will she need permission to leave the bed for any reason (with the obvious exception of emergencies) including going to the bathroom?

The general rule of thumb is that the less you allow her to do during bed arrest, the more effective the punishment. During the sentence master can progressively give her back more privileges, such as no longer needing permission to go to the bathroom, watch TV, play videogames, watch movies, read books, use the phone, etc. Also was she tied to the bed at all times? Maybe now she can be unbound. (I would strongly suggest that except for emergencies she is never allowed to use the phone during bed arrest.)

My experience is that it's best to start the bed arrest with her having as few privileges as possible and being bound securely to the bed. You then give privileges back as she earns them and/or begs enough for them.

As it's likely you will let her out of the bed to fix meals and do other chores, you'll then need to make sure she's not taking unusually long to do those activities. If so master may want to threaten her with extending her sentence or perhaps another good spanking will take care of that problem.

4. Bondage and blindfolding during her incarceration. Will she be tied up and/or tied to the bed in bondage for a significant amount of the sentence? I would suggest she is and for a substantial amount of time, at least in the first half or more of her incarceration. Blindfolds can help make her feel more isolated and increase the impact of the punishment. Master will probably want to tie her hands in manner so that she **can't** take the blindfold off when she thinks master is not looking, or at least lower the blindfold a bit to look around real quick. Obviously a respectful, well trained sub/slave should not do this but sub/slaves are after all human.

5) Sub/slave needing permission from her master to leave the bed for anything (other than emergencies.) It may seem harsh but my experience is that bed arrest as a punishment works best when to leave the bed for even essential activities, such as going to the bathroom, the sub/slave first needs to have permission from her master. Because of this the master will find that he will need to be in the dwelling and at earshot at all times, just incase, which obviously could be inconvenient for him. With good behavior on her part, this restriction can be lessened.

6) Master will always determine what she does or doesn't wear during the period of bed arrest. *(This is of course is subject to how cold it is, if company shows up and/or if she has to go out of the house for work or other essential activities.)*

During bed arrest, while in private, it's suggested that she not be allowed to wear any clothing.

During the period of her incarceration, also perhaps remove her authority to wear panties while she is out of the house/apartment doing essential public activities such as work and shopping. *(Don't be surprised if she won't go along with this, particularly if it entails doing this at work. If that's the case guys, let it go.)*

7) Pouting, sulking and possibly rebelling by the sub/slave. Master should prepare for his sub/slave to possibly pout, sulk, and as a lengthy sentence progresses, maybe even try to rebel, though hopefully without going too far. Of course the more time master spends with her in bed, playing with her, spanking her, taking her being massaged by her, lying in bed with her, the happier she'll likely be but perhaps the punishment will be less effective, (or perhaps it could have just the opposite effect and be of good benefit).

It's possible that she will rebel to the point that she says she hates you and leaves the house frustrated. It is her right guys and you can't stop her, unfortunately it's likely also a sign of problems in the relationship, and/or a poorly trained sub/slave and/or a sub/slave that simply does not allow herself to be punished with bed arrest, (and/or perhaps other punishments you include during bed arrest.)

Still perhaps she has had a bad experience with bed arrest in the past? That will have to be dealt with in a responsible, respectful manner.

What if she doesn't like bondage and/or blindfolding then either she takes the plunge and lets you do that to her or you don't do those activities.

Perhaps she has obligations that she feels will interfere with the length of her sentence. You would need to let her off for those obligations anyway and perhaps she doesn't understand that.

On the other hand you as master might now find out that she is not a respectful sub/slave, an immature sub/slave and/or too much of a bratty sub/slave and you should find another.

8) Adding more time to her sentence as well as commuting her sentence. The sub/slave should be aware that more time can be added to her sentence. Additionally privileges might not be returned to her as fast during her sentence if she continues to be a bad girl and/or doesn't seem to be learning her lesson.

On the other hand, if she displays a respectful attitude and takes her punishment respectfully then the opposite can occur. Time can be taken off her sentence, and privileges can be returned more quickly during her sentence.

9. How often can we play while she is in bed arrest? Well guys, she's tied up to the bed, naked and blindfolded, good luck keeping your hands off of her! Still the master isn't the one being punished here so his needs and pleasure shouldn't suffer. If he wants his sub/slave to massage him, she should massage him. If he wants fellatio from his sub/slave, by all means get it. If he wants to take his slave, by all means take her. Still it breaks the monotony for her which might not be as conducive to punishment. But it will likely will give her pleasure, make her feel more wanted and loved. Hopefully that won't interfere with her learning her lesson and it might in fact help. Perhaps playing with her later during her incarceration is the better choice, if the master can hold out that long.

Hopefully throughout her sentence she will be on her best behavior in an attempt to get her sentence reduced.

10. What activities can the sub/slave do while she is in bed arrest?

A) Of course her work and parental responsibilities are fully allowed. (If you're living with kids, as you can imagine this punishment could be difficult to perform.)

Still master must watch to make sure she doesn't spend more time than she ordinarily would with her responsibilities. When that's the case her master may wish to add time to her incarceration and/or punish her in other ways.

B) She is required to satisfy her master's sexual desires as always as well as any other activities that can be performed on the bed that she would ordinarily do for her master. This includes massaging her master.

C) Her master perhaps may still also want to punish her in one or more other manners.

11. Privileges that can be taken away from the sub/slave during bed arrest include (depending on circumstances):

*Being able to enjoy video entertainment such as playing video games, watching videos, TV, movies, etc. That can include her favorite programming that would come on during her period of incarceration. (It can be recorded to be watched after her sentence is over.)

*Being able to talk (unless there is an emergency) or she needs permission to do something.

*Being able to use the phone.

*Being able to write things by hand.

*Being able to read for entertainment, such as books.

*Being allowed to have orgasms or otherwise pleasure herself (but dude that's harsh!)

12. Do you close the door on her during her confinement? No, but it's the master's choice if she's allowed to look at him.

13. How to react to her begging during incarceration. If your sub/slave is adept at begging and if they can be real sexy while doing it, masters may have to ban begging during bed arrest altogether or deal with the horniness that comes with it.

I for one like it when she begs and you can require a certain number of "begs" from her before you'll even consider commuting her sentence.

14. Additional punishments while she is in bed arrest. Perhaps you would like to give her "hourlies". These are spankings given every hour during a set period. She needs to make sure that her master knows it is time for her hourly spanking (or other prescribed hourly punishment) or risk having addition time added to her sentence.

15. Additional general advice to the master. Guys you need to hold strong and be firm. That can be tough. Make sure she takes you seriously throughout this period.

The End

Book #3 – Dramatic Weight Loss Using BDSM

By Phil G.

Other Books by EroticBDSMbooks.com Include:

The Absolutely Essential Book of BDSM and S&M Rules
Things To Do During 3 Hours of Sex; A Step-by-step Guide
Playtime At The Dom Den; A Step-by-step Guide
The Absolutely Essential Guide to Great BDSM and S&M Sex
The Absolutely Essential Dominant/submissive Playtime Experience
The Absolutely Essential BDSM Sexual Experience
The Ultimate Collection of S&M and BDSM Rules For Female Submissives and Slaves
Master and submissive or slave BDSM Contract
Mistress/slave BDSM Contract
Have Awesome BDSM Sex
BDSM Master/slave Contract
Spanking Dictionary
BDSM Rules
Bed Arrest, the Punishment for BDSM Enthusiasts

Dramatic Weight Loss Using BDSM

Introduction

BDSM is uniquely qualified to help people lose weight. I'm personally familiar with many women who have successfully lost a surprising amount of weight using this system.

If you are not familiar with BDSM (*Bondage, Discipline, Sadism and/or Masochism,*) please do an Internet search or otherwise learn it better (should that be your wish.) This book has been written primarily for those well acquainted with the lifestyle.

As you know losing weight is an arduous, restrictive, sacrifice-filled experience that isn't particularly fun. To fight this, the dieter needs a lot of motivation. Happily BDSM can be of great service regarding that.

In this book, for simplicity's sake, the dieter is going to be a submissive female and the dieting taskmaster is going to be a dominant male (as well as her Dominant.) Obviously the sexes can be reversed, or instead both parties can be the same sex.

Integral to successful weight loss using BDSM is that the dieter needs to be submissive to the Dominant and relinquish control to him of those aspects of her life that affect her weight loss, such as her dieting. (Case studies are presented later in this book.)

As a Master I have overseen many female submissive/slave's BDSM weight loss programs, and often with very good success. There is no doubt that this kind of BDSM weight loss program can be a first rate weight loss plan. It has proven itself many times.

The biggest problems however are that the dieter (the submissive):

(a) Decides against continuing with the restrictions of the weight loss program (such as the diet)
(b) Rebels against the dominance of her Dominant. (If this occurs, likely all is lost.)

Talk to each other about this in the beginning and again as necessary. Be prepared for it so you can talk about it when (and if) it occurs.

In this weight loss program the dominant will exercise strict control over what she (the submissive) eats and will punish her for infractions as he feels is necessary. She can't rebel against this or the weight loss program likely won't succeed.

She also needs to be honest with herself and to her Dom. She can't go about eating foods (or excess amounts of food) that she isn't allowed to, and/or lie about it, etc. Should she fail regarding this, she should be punished and she needs to accept that.

Unfortunately during the BDSM Weight Loss Program one or more of these problems can manifest themselves:

A) Life throws her a curve ball and she (the dieter) has to get off the weight loss program. In that case let it go and restart it ASAP.

B) Women just don't like to be told they're overweight no matter how true it is, so even discussing it can be a sensitive subject, and that includes while the BDSM Weight Loss Program is going on! *It's very helpful if the woman works past this as it's natural during this time to think that her Dominant has a negative view of her current possibly overweight body.*

I can think of a particular time I put a slave on a BDSM weight loss program and she rebelled after only around 6 days. I'm confident it was not my fault. We ended up ending our online relationship because of this. I was in contact with her a couple of months later and happily she had restarted dieting and had lost a significant amount of weight.

Even though it was me who had finally inspired *and required* her to get on a weight loss program of any sort, she did not in any way associate her weight-loss success with me anymore at that point (and unfairly in my opinion.)

C) The Dominant is not good at this and the submissive needs to break it off due to that. Perhaps he's not a good Dom to start out with or she doesn't respect him as much as both had thought she did. (It helps if the Dom is in decent physical shape and exercises himself but that is comparatively minor.)

The Dominant needs to know how much (and how hard) to push her but if she is sensitive to this type of control then the program is likely doomed to failure.

D) She doesn't want to lose weight bad enough.

E) She rebels against certain specific demands of this strict regimen.

Beware dominants, as previously noted, your relationship with this submissive can readily end because of enforcing the BDSM Weight Loss Program. If she gives up on the program the Dominant can push her to continue but at some point he had best give up or the relationship will almost certainly suffer. I have lost more than one lady because I didn't give up fast enough (though actually it was more because she gave up on the weight loss program too quickly in my opinion.)

What To Do To Implement The
BDSM Weight Loss Program

A) To start out with, the submissive needs to accept that she needs to lose weight. (Hopefully she adamantly wants to lose weight.) The other option is that her Dom/Domme has told her to and she is going to obey him.

B) She might first try the usual methods of losing and keeping weight off, and hopefully that works. If those attempts aren't fruitful enough, or if she wants to try another type of weight loss program from the get-go, then the *BDSM Weight Loss Program* is definitely a way to go.

C) If possible, determine just what the weight loss program's specifics will be. It doesn't need to be complex or extreme.

BDSM weight loss typically is a combination of exercise, good sleep, an acceptable level of stress and diet/calorie restrictions. The more sex she can have during this time, typically the better. Does she have a convenient way to exercise? Does she know where to get low calorie food?

The lack of optimal gut microbes have been tentatively linked to many overweight people are so perhaps a probiotic should be taken but beware, most, if not all of the live bacteria in a probiotic supplement is killed by stomach acid so get one that can best survive stomach acid on its way to the colon where it has important work to do. Low calorie yogurt has at least somewhat of a probiotic effect.

D) Can she afford Nutrisystems, Jenny Craig, Weight Watchers, Medifast or something of that nature? If so you'll likely want to go with that.

E) Does she understand nutrition well enough to know the allowable foods to eat? Most women do. If not her Dom will have to have even stricter control over the food she eats.

F) Tell the sub/slave on what day the program begins. Give her at least one day to party a bit and experience the culinary freedom that she won't have for some time.

G) Maintenance spankings can be a good idea during the weight loss program. This helps the submissive's conscious and/or subconscious mind remember the importance of respecting her commitment to the program and the authority of her Dom who will oversee it and punish her (and reward her) when she fails to keep her end of the bargain.

Definition of a Maintenance Spanking: Spankings administered on a regular basis to keep the spankee on the straight and narrow. (Punishment spankings are administered in addition to these.)

H) Provide encouragement for the submissive and perhaps give her extra time to work out by doing certain chores that take up her time and/or energy.

I) At some point down the road she can start increasing her calorie intake but that should be after significant weight loss or if there are health issues.

J) In most cases it's helpful for weight loss if she speeds up her metabolism in some healthy way.

K) Important, don't forget about rewarding her for her weight loss accomplishments. Be liberal with the rewards. She'll likely really appreciate those and rewards may be the difference in the success or failure of her adherence to the program. I personally would not include higher calorie treats as a reward but it's up to you. The truth is that the sub/slave typically will really look forward to her rewards (though the bigger ones need to be substantial, like a night out or a new special article of clothing, etc.) The sub/slave should feel free to remind her Dom about the rewards from time to time and if the Dom is not rewarding her in a noticeable and significant manner, it's my opinion that he is not keeping up his end of the bargain.

Be generous with minor rewards like watching something she wants to on TV or fixing a nice low calorie dinner for her if the Dom doesn't normally do that. Throw in bigger rewards periodically. Perhaps it is she who should choose, or at least recommend the upcoming reward. (I think it can be better when it is she who chooses at least the major rewards.)

Rule: Rewards <u>cannot</u> be taken away as punishment. She has to be able to take her punishment like a good girl and once she's been punished, it's over. The slate has been wiped clean because she paid fully for her transgression thanks to the punishment. I for one will only supervise a BDSM Weight Loss Program where I can punish her at will. Having a corner to send her to stand in after her well deserved spanking is also a great idea! (If she won't let you spank her then I suspect this weight loss program is not for you two, or it's a long distance relationship.)

Getting her a new sex toy(s) can be a good reward. (As a Dom I require my slave to have a huge amount of sexual pleasure from playing so new sex toys work nicely.)

As a reward, periodically you should take her out to eat where she can have a moderate calorie meal.

L) *Compliments* – We all know how much women love compliments. Doms, don't forget to compliment her for her hard work regarding the weight loss program.

It will also be very helpful if she has a dieting and/or workout support system with family and/or friends. Two or more women starting a weight loss program together is often a great thing, maybe even throw in a bet as to who would be the first to quit.

Perhaps the Dom and sub/slave would like to do this together, both going on at least a diet. A problem is that the Dom can't get punished as readily for transgressions (or can he?) Perhaps he can lower his calorie intake out of respect for what she's going through particularly if they live together.

Her overweight friends and family that don't want to deal with the concept of weight loss can be a problem. They might tell her she looks fine and that she shouldn't feel she needs to work out and/or diet due to their own insecurity and/or laziness. That position however is not good for our situation.

Rules for the Submissive During the
BDSM Weight Loss Program

1) The dieter will report specifics (via email or phone) *every* night as to what she ate that day/night and what weight loss activities she engaged in. (It's kind of a diary.) As is obvious, this way her Dom can better keep an eye on her activities.

2) If she wants to eat more than a heaping tablespoon of any higher calorie food, she MUST first get permission from her Dom. (*Her Dom needs to give examples of what "higher calorie food" is.*) For example, if there is an unexpected office party and cake is served, she would need to steal away and call up her Dom and ask permission to have a small slice. (To review, up to a heaping tablespoon in a multi-hour time period never needs permission. More than that *always* needs permission.)

3) Skipping workouts (assuming workouts are part of the program, which ideally they should be) are not allowed unless she has an excellent excuse. (Having a stationary bicycle and/or Stairmaster type of exercise device where she lives can work very well and is convenient. Often thrift stores have these.) **To skip a workout, or not to workout hard enough, she needs permission from her Dom unless there is a health issue**. If she misses a workout for a less than suitable reason, or her workouts are not of an acceptable nature and/or intensity, *she should be punished*!

4) To the Doms reading this, during a lasting weight loss program your resolve will almost certainly be tested by your submissive and you must be prepared to follow through with the threat of punishment, unless she has a good excuse or there are health concerns.

It's very important that she respect you as the administrator of the weight loss program and enforcer of the weight loss program's admittedly arduous restrictions.

It is also a rule that she must accept her punishment.

If you announce a punishment and she balks then chances are either the punishment is unreasonable or she just isn't ready for weight loss the BDSM way.

5) If the dieter has health concerns then the weight loss program is at least suspended. All health concerns must be taken seriously and addressed immediately!

Case Study #1

Lori started the BDSM weight loss program under my guidance. She formerly was my slave (but wasn't at that time.) She still had a strong respect for me as a Dominant though and we played semi-regularly. (As amazing as it sounds, I'm proud to say we actually had an amicable break-up. Yes amicable break-ups really can happen!)

Day #1 – During the previous day she partier with her son. That night she had a sugary soft drink, several slices of regular pizza, salad from the salad bar with a very generous helping of higher calorie salad dressing. Later they had ice cream cones.

The program started the next day with weighing herself after defecating (but before eating.)

Lori could afford Nutrisystem, had preordered and was able to start eating those that day. She had a stationary bicycle in her living room.

We did not live together but were in the same vicinity so we could see each other in person without too much trouble (especially since I lived alone and was self-employed.)

That day she only ate Nutrisystems meals and exercised on the stationary bike for 10 minutes. (She hadn't used the stationary bike in a while.)

We talked on the phone that night and she reported what she ate and told me about her workout. Clearly it was an excellent start for her.

Day #2-4: Nothing eventful. She kept to the plan and reported every night what she did in regard to exer-cycling, walking around the neighborhood and eating. As she was eating Nutrisystems it was easier for her to report her meals. She just needed to say "Nutrisystem meals".

Day #5: She had gone out that night with girlfriends and had 2 Kuala's with crème (the very tasty alcoholic beverage.) This was a problem as she at least needed to call me to ask permission to have the second higher than normal calorie drink, which she didn't. (Frankly having a lower calorie alcoholic beverage would have been better.)

I explained to her how what she did was wrong (which she knew) and had her come over to my place the next day for punishment.

Now is an important time. She might take more diet damaging liberties if her subconscious doesn't realize she can't get away with it. So punishment it would be and frankly it turned us both on anyway☺

I waited alone in my house and she came over while her son was in school. As was standard with us, she was only allowed to wear a skirt or dress when we're together (this dress I picked out for her over the phone last night.) As usual, upon entering she was required to remove her panties and leave them in a dresser by the door. (None of my slaves are allowed to wear panties in my home except for emergencies and when leaving.) She knelt down in front of me and I proceeded to scold her for not abiding by the diet rules. I opened her dress top and played with her breasts while she promised to be good and apologized. I then had her stand up and remove her dress, then kneel down again so I could tie her hands together. She was ordered to lie across my lap so I could give her a good spanking. I used a strap, a slapper and a small paddle and reddened her butt nicely. She made yelps, squirmed and kicked her feet. I then ordered her to stand in the corner, periodically coming over and spanking her while she was there. She once again promised to adhere to the rules. I then ordered her into the bedroom where we had sex and otherwise played for several hours. During our playtime her hands remained tied together.

It was that day that I instigated maintenance spankings every 3 days (if convenient for her, though sometimes it wasn't as we didn't live together and she lived with her son as a single mother.)

Day #6 – Lori's morning weigh in showed she had lost 3 pounds since beginning the diet. She was real happy about it. I thought I saw a difference in her yesterday and had told her that. She called during lunch and wanted to know if she could have the lasagna for lunch at the restaurant but I wouldn't allow it.

That night she emailed me what she ate and drank that day. She also described her workout. She said that she worked out at home with her 7 year old son and they had a good time working out together.

Day #7 – Nothing eventful.

Day #8 – Lori comes over for a maintenance spanking and of course we have sex. Like my punishment spankings her bottom is made red, though not as red as a punishment spanking. I use a variety of spanking implements too. (It's always been my rule that a slave has no more than 60 seconds to be wet from a spanking. No spanking even has the chance of ending until she's wet [with the exception of emergencies of course.])

Lori could take a hard spanking so the red bottom I would make sure to give her before the spanking was over, might be too hard for some other ladies to take. Lori remembered fondly how a paddle broke on her butt at a spanking party.

Day #9 – Lori reports that the dress she initially put on for work was loose, loose enough to make her feel uncomfortable. She had forgotten to weigh herself before eating breakfast so no new weigh-in but we anticipated good news. She sent an email late that night jokingly noting the heaping tablespoon of her son's ice cream she had. She wrote that her workout was 20 minutes on the stationary bicycle and it made her work up a good sweat.

Day #10 – Lori weighs herself after defecating and has lost 6 pounds since beginning the diet. At work already her weight loss was getting noticed and compliments were being handed out. When people ask her how she was doing it she just said

Nutrisystems and exercising, primarily on her stationary bicycle. (It could get her in trouble at work to bring up the BDSM thing.)

Day #11 – This is maintenance spanking day but Lori couldn't get a babysitter so it didn't happen. She was in a bad mood though and my frustration about her not coming over upset her. Fortunately I soothed things over before the conversation ended.

Day #12 – Lori calls that night and wants to eat a small slice of her sister's peach pie which I let her do. She forgot to send me the nightly email report. I told her to come over for punishment ASAP. She apologized and tried to get a babysitter but couldn't find one until two nights later on day #14.

Day #13 – I realized I had not rewarded her yet with anything significant (actually she reminded me over the phone) and I felt bad. The next night she had her babysitter and we went to a Native American casino and I gave her $50 to gamble with, after our meal at the buffet. (As you can imagine I watched her like a hawk as she took food.) We got back to my place and I gave her the maintenance spanking she very much needed, leaving her lovely bare bottom a beautiful shade of red. We had sex of course.

Day #14-15 – Nothing eventful.

Day #16 – Lori weigh-in showed she'd lost a total of 9 pounds and frankly her weight loss for a woman in her 30s was even better than anyone expected. She voiced concern about her dwindling clothing supply (that would fit well.) She began wearing skirts and blouses more which made her feel sexier and seemed to adapt better to her shrinking body. She was being noticed in a positive way at work and got the impression it made her look like someone that can get things done, has drive and has follow-through.

She was a bit frustrated by her somewhat shrinking boobs but the shrinkage was minor. The fact was that she had become a darn good advertisement for Nutrisystems and even her mother planned to start using them. (This book however does not necessarily recommend them over other weight loss nutrition programs.)

Little did anyone other than us know that it was also the *BDSM Weight Loss Program* that was working so well, particularly in providing motivation.

Day #17 – She forgot to email me her daily food and activities. I promise to ad an addition 30 spanks during her next maintenance spanking for that.

Day #18 – With her son gone out of town to his grandmother's for the weekend I was able to spend the night over at her place. I give her her maintenance spanking that evening and have a good time playing with her. I blindfolded her and tied her to the bed in tight bondage and left her there for over an hour. I spanked her again and took her as she laid there helplessly tied up.

After finally releasing her, we showered together and she made us a late dinner of which she also ate instead of nutrisystem food. It was Chop suey filled with vegetables. She had around a cup of rice and a good helping of the Chop suey.

The next morning we got up late, I got stuck with a honey-do list of stuff to do at her place which I spent 6 hours doing, then we played. That night we went through all her cloths to see which no longer "looked good" on her due to the weight loss. (I frankly thought more of her cloths looked fine on her than she did.)

We weeded out about 30% of her cloths and put the cloths that she thought were too big in a separate side of the closet. (Happily her sister had a lot of cloths that would fit Lori's progressively more petite body. Her sister had grown out of those several years ago.)

Well I guess now I'll wrap up my report on Lori. Lori did extremely well on the BDSM weight loss diet. I attribute it to these factors:

1) She really wanted to lose weight; it was an obsession to her.
2) Her body could lose weight faster than many other folks. Perhaps she had a faster metabolism.

3) She had been into BDSM for over 6 years and was very comfortable with her role as a slave.

4) She respected me very much as a Dominant and frankly I again became more of a Master to her. I even collared her on day 23. It was another reward for her doing so well.

5) I did a good job as the Dominant. I backed down in more than one occasion where there could have been trouble if I pushed too much harder. I did a good job with her and frankly I can't say that about all the sub/slaves I administered BDSM Weight Loss with.

6) She also relished all the attention and kudos she got and wasn't hurt that much from the jealousy that more overweight women projected on her.

7) She could afford a specialized nutritional program such as Nutrisystems, Jenny Craig, Weight Watchers, Medifast, etc.

8) She wasn't a food addict and did fine not eating that much even when she was around others that were eating.

Case Study #2

Michele was mostly an online/phone slave of mine. She lived about 260 miles away. I pushed her to start the BDSM weight loss program under my guidance as she was overweight. She wasn't my slave but respected me as a Dominant.

Michelle didn't have Nutrisystems or something of that nature so she would have to concentrate on buying low calorie foods. She did however have a fitness club membership that she had paid for but stopped using.

She drove over to my place for the weekend. She got there Friday night and stayed through Sunday afternoon. Saturday is when the BDSM Weight Loss Program started.

We played throughout the weekend and I made sure she did most of the work screwing. She was out of shape but really worked hard during sex which no doubt burned a lot of calories. Of course I kept her bottom well spanked throughout the weekend. I personally think the sub/slave being well spanked helps the weight loss program but I may be wrong.

We spent a good deal of time setting up her meals. We went online to get ideas and got a huge list of low calorie things for her to make. (Of course there are all the pre-made diet TV dinners to buy in the store.)

Something we tried was having her drink A LOT of water to try and fill her stomach up thus countering hunger pains. That had mixed results.

I had a Stairmaster at my house and made her walk and even run on it twice on Saturday and Sunday. While she was naked on the Stairmaster, I stood behind her with a paddle and paddled her when she didn't walk/run fast enough. As previously noted I made her do as much of the work as possible when we had sex and that included sucking on my cock *many times* each day!

While she was with me she was a very good girl but after she left I could only hope she would obey the rules. She planned on visiting me every other weekend so I could see her progress and punish her in person for not adhering to the rules.

Day #3 – She called to complain about how sore she was from our playtime but also to note what she ate.

Day #4 – Nothing eventful. She sent me the nightly email as to what she ate. She said she was still too sore to go to the gym.

Day #5 – Michelle went to her fitness facility and worked out, mostly working her lower body out. I am sad to report however that Michelle called and admitted to eating two donuts today during a work break. She said she was hungry and just couldn't help herself. Being so far away can make punishment difficult and her next visit was a week and a half away. I feared that she would break down and once again too readily eat forbidden foods. I decided she needed to be punished for that now, as well as when she got here.

One always has to wonder how a particular sub/slave will take to being scolded/punished as she could become defensive and call the whole thing off (if that happens then most likely she was not a good candid for successful BDSM weight loss anyway.) I told her that her punishment for now is that she's not allowed to wear panties until further notice. Obviously this meant she could not wear a dress or skirt in public but she usually didn't anyway. Also I would tack on an extra, good spanking with the paddle when she next came to visit. Before she hung up though I told her she could wear panties for her excursions to the fitness club.

Day #6 – Michelle had weighed herself after defecating (and before eating of course) and had lost 3 pounds since the start of the diet. She emailed me the good news! She also told me how she was at work with no panties on, which excited me. I emailed back congratulating her about the weight loss and told her to report what life is like while not wearing panties. That night she called. She told me of her now panty-less life and gave me the report as to what she ate that day, which was very little, so little that I voiced my concern.

Day #7 – Michelle called that evening and wanted to know if she could have a chicken pasta dish at the restaurant she was at with two of her girlfriends. I told her no. She responded to me with silence and I asked her sternly if "she understood young lady?" and she responded with "Yes Sir" and that was that. She later said that one of her girlfriends gave her a hard time for not "splurging" and getting it. Little did her girlfriend know that she wasn't allowed to do it by her "Dom". (To play it safe, it wasn't something Michelle was telling them about either.)

Unfortunately for Michelle, most of her girlfriends had bad eating habits and didn't really care what they looked like. Only one was attractive to start out with. It ended up being a tough night to hang out with her girlfriends. She went home feeling lonely. She called me up and told me of her frustration. I had to give her a pep talk and we had phone sex. I also had to remind her that she had made a commitment to the weight loss program and me, her Dom and she was required to follow through with the commitment. She agreed and felt better. She asked if she could start wearing panties again and I said yes.

(Interestingly the next day one of her girlfriends called and said that Michelle had inspired her and she also was going to try and lose weight, starting with dieting.)

Day #8 – Michelle had gotten into eating raw vegetables with low calorie salad dressing. She also drank pure fruit juice and went to her fitness club to work out. She however forgot to send me her nightly report of what she ate and did for weight loss. She did however the next morning before she went to work (she worked that Saturday) and so I let it slide.

Day #9 – She called to chat and sounded like she was having a lazy Sunday. I was busy and said she should go work out and call me back when she returned. A few hours later she did but she sounded irritable. I finally asked her if she was feeling okay and/or if she was mad about something. She finally said that it frustrated her that I didn't want her the way she was and it seemed that I would only want her if she was the slender "Barbie doll type".

Well this took me by surprise but this is a common way for the lady in the BDSM weight loss program to act and feel, at least periodically.

The truth was I wanted her to look better and be more sexy, the way that more slender women often are. Was I to be blamed for that? The truth was that as a guy I wanted her to be truly height weight proportionate, which she wasn't yet. For some reason I was however not allowed to think that way or was not allowed to take those thoughts seriously. (I certainly was not allowed to voice this desire.)

I had been here before and had told the truth to women which was that I would find her more attractive if she was a more optimal weight, but that offended the women and the relationship always had ended, at least for purposes of the BDSM Weight Loss Program.

Guys now is the time for you to perhaps swallow your pride and perhaps tell a little "white lie", that being that you thought she was just as attractive and desirable now as she would be when she became height weight proportionate, or better yet slender. She wants to hear that and her shot at serious weight loss from the BDSM diet could be lost if you don't.

The truth is I have a good deal of experience administering the BDSM Weight Loss Program and this obstacle comes up *a lot*.

I told Michelle that she just wasn't all she could be and I took this weight loss program very seriously and she should also. It was being done for *her*. I also told her what a fine person she was and that I was sexually attracted to her.

I don't know if she believed me but the phone conversation ended in a somewhat tense manner. I never heard from her that night with her nightly report though and neither of us communicated with each other for a number of days.

Her BDSM Weight Loss Program was over as was our romantic relationship.

Epilogue

The premise of the weight loss program is pretty straight forward. How long she stays with the program is another story.

Both parties should be prepared for the additional competition for her affections that can come into play as she loses weight.

Best of luck to all.

The End

These books are sold and/or distributed with the understanding that the publisher and author is not engaged in rendering legal or other professional services. **These books and their subject matter are for entertainment purposes only.** In these publications there may be inadvertent inaccuracies including technical inaccuracies, typographical inaccuracies and other possible inaccuracies. **The writer and publisher of these publications expressly disclaim all liability for the use or interpretation by anybody of information contained in this publication.** The author, publisher and distributors of this publication hereby disclaim any and all liability for any loss or damage caused by errors or omissions resulted from negligence, accident, or any other causes. If legal advice or other expert assistance is required, the services of a competent professional person in a consultation capacity should be sought. Products, services and websites' content vary with time. Please verify any published information.

Book #4 – The Spanking Dictionary

By Phil G.

Copyright (C) 2013

The Spanking Dictionary

Caution is always advised in anything related to spanking, discipline and punishment. Always stay within legal boundaries.

Spanking pronouns, (which include names of spanking websites, spanking actors/actresses, spanking parties and spanking media) are NOT included in this dictionary due to space limitations. **Spanking of minors is not discussed in this book nor advocated.**

ADULT SPANKING - Spanking taking place among and between people who are of legal age.

ADULT SPANKING SCENARIOS - Spanking activities that take place among adults. These are often thought up and set up ahead of time.

AMATEUR SPANKING – (1) Unless a person is spanking, or receiving spankings for money or other material gain (such as Spanking Therapists and professional FemDoms do,) then this category includes most in the adult spanking world. (2) While not all agree on this angle of the definition, it has been used to imply a spanker or spankee who is not proficient in the spanking arts.

ANAL EXAM – The dominant spends a lot of time inspecting, testing and ultimately using the spankee's anus for his/her pleasure.

ANGER MANAGEMENT THERAPY SPANKING - Spanking can be used as a kind of therapy to help manage anger. There are two different approaches.

(1) The angered/stressed person is the *spankee* and gets spanked for a length and an intensity that allows the anger/stress to be released. Multiple spankings may be needed.

(2) The angered/stressed person is the *spanker* and spanks for a length and an intensity that allows the anger/stress to be released. Multiple spankings may be needed.

ANNIVERSARY SPANKING - Like birthday spankings this involves a tradition where as part of the festivities one or multiple participants spank and/or get spanked. It may include a special sexual scenario also. Spankophiles might want to get creative and have these anniversaries occur on other anniversaries such as when the couple met, became engaged and/or had their first date.

AVERAGE SPANKING (An) – Your basic everyday spanking, the usual. (Yawn.)

BARE BOTTOM SPANKINGS – Applying the spanking directly to the uncovered buttocks.
There are advantages to this versus spanking the covered buttocks:

1) *Better access*; the spanker may wish to use the spankee's bottom for other types of stimulation including anal and vaginal stimulation. The spanker may want to rub the naked bottom sensually at various times, etc.

2) *Humiliation*; the spankee must expose him/herself.

3) *Intensity*; clothing can lessen the impact of the blows and thus lessen the spanking's sensation and/or ability to provide punishment.

4) *Safety*; All parties can see how the buttocks is fairing from the blows. Perhaps the intensity needs to be lessened; you might not know if the buttocks are covered.

BARE BOTTOM BEATING – See *Bare Bottom Spankings*.

BATHBRUSH – A long handled brush used for washing one's self during bathing. It can be an effective spanking tool.

BEDROOM TIME – Being banished to the bedroom after, and/or as part of a punishment spanking. Often this bad girl will get spanked more than once while serving bedroom time.

BED ARREST – A type of BDSM punishment. See *"Bed Arrest, the Punishment for BDSM Enthusiasts"*.

BEDTIME SPANKING – (1) Spankings irregularly administered as foreplay to sex prior to going to sleep for the night. (2) Spankings which are administered nightly (or irregularly) when the spankee and/or spanker goes to bed, whether there is to be sexual activity or not.

A number of spankees claim a bedtime spanking helps make them sleepy.

BEHAVIOR MODIFICATION SPANKING – Spanking(s) administered to change unwanted behavior. Repeated and hard spankings may well be necessary to make this work.

BELT – It holds a man's pants up and is a nasty spanking implement. You're in for it now young lady!

BIRCHING – Birching is to spank using a tied together collection of thin tree switches. A nice touch is to have the spankee go out and pick the tree switches herself and tie them together securely for future use or use as soon as it is made.

BIRTHDAY SPANKING - A "traditional" birthday spanking is given on the birthday of the spankee. The formula is to administer one swat for each year of age, plus one additional swat "to grow on, one to live on, one to be happy on, to get married on, etc." The last swat can be the hardest as it's for any bad behavior that he/she did last year.

Spankee beware! Many will say that each birthday party attendee gets to give the same number of spanks, which can make for hundreds of spanks!

The spankee might pick and choose who gets to do the spanking and birthday spankings are typically done clothed as it's often done at children's parties.

Birthday spankings are usually done by hand but if it involves consenting adults spanking that often won't be the case.

Dominants may want to incorporate "practice birthday spankings" with their submissives as another excuse to spank.

Birthday spankings can be given belatedly but typically are for only the spankee's previous birthday (not all his/her birthdays.)

Blindfolding the adult spankee might be a nice touch.

A *"Reverse Birthday Spanking"* is when the person having the birthday gets to give the spankings instead!

BOARD OF CORRECTION – Slang name for a paddle.

BOTTOMS UP – While more known as a saying for drinking everything from a glass (container) so the bottom of the container is pointing up (thus sending all the liquid into your mouth,) this also means presenting a bottom for a spanking.

BOTTOM RAKING - Sliding your fingernails over and across the spanked or unspanked ass. This should not be done hard enough to puncture the skin or even take any layers of skin off. This should also only be done over the fleshy part of the buttocks and not near the anus or sexual organs.

BROKE THE PADDLE ON MY BUTT – This saying can be put in different ways. It's a source of pride for the spankee that when someone spanked his/her butt using a paddle, the paddle broke upon hitting his/her butt.

BRUTAL SPANKING – See *Severe Spanking*.

CAPSAICIN CREAM – (Results vary from individual to individual.) - Applying a *very small* amount of this cream onto the naked buttocks is an alternative to spanking (thus is called *"Silent Spanking"*). It seeps into the bottom and often is painful. A surprisingly small amount is needed. Make sure to quickly wash your hands after applying it or you will be in pain too. (Better yet use something else to apply it with.)

Rub the *capsaicin cream* in well. It might take some time to make its impact well noticed. Spankers I suggest you first experiment by rubbing a tiny bit into your spankee's butt. Only drops of it would be necessary to first test his/her resistance to it. Olive oil or vegetable oil can help dissipate the pain. This cream may look innocent but the stuff is *evil*! (Tiger Balm is another possible punishment cream.) Do not put any of this on or in the anus or vagina!

CANING – This is when a cane is applied with force to the buttocks of the spankee. The cane can hurt more than many other spanking implements due to its smaller surface area so caution is advised. Also see *Switching*.

CARPET BEATER – A long handled housekeeping tool used to beat dust off of hanging rugs and to spank worthy bottoms.

CHARITY SPANKING - Charity Spanking is when people are spanked in exchange for others sponsoring them and giving money to one or more charities for each good spank they take. Also see *Professional Spanking*.

CLENCHING – (Clenching Cheeks) – This is when the spankee tightens his/her buttocks muscles together forcefully. This might be done in an attempt to dull the sting of the spanking.

COMING BACK IN FROM THE PUBLIC SPANKINGS – After the spankee returns to a private secluded setting, after having been in the public (and that includes having been to work or having been shopping), she gets a spanking as a natural course of events. This is over and above any other spankings she's getting for any other reason. This is associated with but the opposite of *Going Out in the Public Spanking*.

CONFESSIONAL {THERAPY} SPANKING - (1) A religiously related spanking scene where the spanker plays an authoritative person of religious faith who spanks the spankee in an effort to get him/her to be more religiously righteous or pay for his/her sins. This may be more popular in Domestic Discipline households. (This happened for real a lot more in centuries past than most hear about.)

(2) The spankee perhaps was raised in a strict religious environment and needs that type of strict (and perhaps regular) guidance to stay on the straight and narrow. A good spanking once or twice a week for just this could be a pleasant addition to your relationship. This obviously has similarities to the confessional of Catholics and doing penance.

(3) In an attempt to get the spankee to confess to something, he/she is spanked. Once he/she confesses then punishment would be administered, which would be another type of spanking such as *Punishment Spanking.*

CONFIDENTIAL SPANKING – The spanking partners agree to keep their spanking relationship and other spanking related activities secret, except to whom they both agree on. It is essential to follow this rule.

CONSENSUAL SPANKING – Informed and agreed-upon spanking that takes place between and among consenting adults.

CORPORAL PUNISHMENT – This is physical punishment inflicted on the human body. This includes spanking but can also include the death penalty.

CROP – A slapping instrument originally meant to urge horses to move. It can be a wonderful spanking implement.

CRUEL TO BE KIND – A saying that is loosely associated with the potentially beneficial impact of adult spanking.

DETENTION ROOM – This is where many naughty schoolgirls go in spanking films and fantasies. This is the location of much discipline, primarily spanking.

DISCIPLINARIAN – Someone with authority that dispenses discipline, often by giving spankings.

DISCIPLINE - It incorporates punishment to correct disobedience of the rules and/or other unacceptable behavior.

DIZZY SPANKING - For this kind of spanking, the spankee is spun around on foot or in a chair that can spin around, until he/she is dizzy. The spankee is then spanked. This is for healthy spankees only and it's essential to take care for safety.

DOMESTIC DISCIPLINE – (*Christian Domestic Discipline, Spanking for Jesus, Loving Domestic Discipline*) – This typically is discipline relegated for couples, and often is administered in Christian dominated households. Rules are instituted and penalties for disobedience are administered. The male tends to be the dominate person (*Head of Household* [HOH]).

DOMINATION SPANKING – The spanking often includes additional aspects of domination such as oral commands, punishment and physical restraint.

DROPSEAT PAJAMAS – These pajamas open at the buttocks for excreting waste and spanking.

DUEL SPANKING - (*Tandem Spanking*) - This is a *Spanking Contest* between spanking couples. The spanking is done simultaneous or one at a time. See *Spanking Contest*.

ENDURANCE SPANKING - This can be done to determine the spanking length and intensity limits of a spankee. (Of course limits change with time.) How much can the spankee take, how many swats, how hard can the swats be, how long can the spanking go on? Are there certain spanking implements that the spankee doesn't do as well with?

Spanking models often go through this unless they have good references.

ENEMA SPANKINGS – Combining enemas with spankings. The spankee is given a spanking then an enema is administered. The spankee releases the water and immediately gets another spanking.

EROTIC SPANKING - Erotic Spanking are spanking activities and techniques that are executed expressly to enhance sexual pleasure. Admittedly spanking (even the thought of spanking) likely enhances a spankopile's pleasure but with *Erotic Spanking* it's taken a step further. For instance the couple can alternate spankings with the use of a variety of sexual toys and/or manual sexual stimulation.

The spankee can be securely tied down so she/he is immobile and can be enjoyed in other ways after and in-between spankings.

EXERCISE SPANKING – If the spankee needs motivation to exercise and/or exercise harder, spanking can be of use. The spankee can be spanked whenever exercise goals are not reached and/or can get the more desirable reward of a pleasurable spanking when the goals are met.

EXHIBITION SPANKING – This is when spanking models, professional or amateur, provide the public with a spanking related show. The spankee(s) could be clothed or exposed. Also see *Public Spanking*.

EXORCISM SPANKING – ("Exorcism Beating") - This occurred historically in various places and times in both western and eastern orthodox Christianity, as well as in other religions. This also occurred as part of the inquisitions. In most cases however, the spankee was lucky if their main punishment was only being spanked (beaten.)

Over the centuries some clergy members, particularly those that still were allowed to have sex, set up chambers where women were spanked, sometimes on a sizable wooden cross, for their purported transgressions. It might have been just one spanking or a semi-regular occurrence.

The spankee's buttocks may or may not be exposed for the beating and onlookers may or may not be allowed to watch, or even aid in the beatings.

F/f SPANKING – Female spanking female.

F/m SPANKING - Female spanking male.

FIFTY SHADES OF GREY - A groundbreaking, famous 2011 erotic romance novel by British author E. L. James. Its erotic scenes include BDSM activities such as bondage, discipline, dominance/submission, sadism and masochism.

FIRM HAND – The spanker has a strong and likely big hand that can deliver impressively hard spanks.

FLOGGING – A flogger is a variation of the cat-of-nine-tails whip. It's typically made of suede or real leather and has many individual elastic strands attached to the handle.

GOING OUT IN THE PUBLIC SPANKING – Before the spankee goes out into the public (and that includes going to work or shopping), she gets a spanking as a natural course of events. This is over and above any other spankings she's getting for any other reason. This is associated with *Coming Back in from the Public Spankings*.

GOOD OLD FASHION SPANKING – These are the standard spankings we grew up with. *Silent Spankings* and many if not all spankings when the spanker is tied down to spanking furniture, likely are not in this category. This term denotes a hard or harder than normal spanking.

GROUP SPANKING – When a multiplicity of people conjugate for the expressed purposes of engaging in one or more kinds of spanking and spanking related endeavors.

HALLOWEEN SPANKING – Spanking on Halloween while people are in costume. Ideally the spankee(s) should not know who's doing the spanking. Another version has it that the spankee(s) are the ones that people can't tell the identity of.

HAIRBRUSH – (Hated Hairbrush) – The household hairbrush makes a very effective and surprisingly intense spanking tool. Mmmmmm!

HAND SPANKING – Directly applying the spanking blows to those naughty butt cheeks with your hand(s).

HANDPRINT – On a well spanked red ass, if the spanker lands a single hard spank, a white handprint on the otherwise red ass cheek might appear for a short time.

HARD SPANKINGS – A true spankophile should be able to take a hard spanking, at least from time to time. Hard spankings might only be relegated for punishment. Technically a hard spanking should not have the intensity of a severe spanking. Depending however on the pain threshold level of the spankee, a hard spanking could make a spankee cry.

Hard spankings however may evolve into your norm. You may find it best to tie down the spankee for a hard spanking.

The spanker can make demands of the spankee during a hard spanking, demands that need to be promised to be met before the spanking can stop. Perhaps by using a vibrator in her anus she would be required to cum before the spanking could stop.

Unless the spankee has very developed resistance, his/her bottom should be red and perhaps marked from a hard spanking.

If the spankee is female it's suggested that no hard spanking ever ends unless her pussy is wet just from the spanking and she's promising to be a very good girl!

HEATING PAD – (1) After a good spanking, if additional punishment is warranted, laying the heated pad over the well spanked buttocks might be the answer. (2) The spankee could place his/her butt on the heating pad before the spanking possibly making it more tender. (3) For some sitting on the heating pad can feel like punishment.

HOLIDAY SPANKING – Spankings in some cases can really add to the holiday cheer! (Of course there's always *Spanking Santa* in his red outfit!)

HOT SPANKING – Spanking that are more sexually stimulating than most.

HOUSE PADDLE – A paddle that is kept readily available as a courtesy for guests to use. (It can be another spanking implement instead and named accordingly).

HUMILIATION THERAPY SPANKING – Sometimes a person needs more humility, one way to give him or her more humility is to combine domination with long, hard spankings. Or just a long hard spanking could do the trick. Spanking Therapists and FemDoms can specialize in this.

ICE SPANKING – There are variations to this spanking technique. If you're interested you and your partner should experiment and find the way that works best for you.

The spankee will need to have her buttocks fully exposed. The spanker can do any of the following, or combine them:

a) First rub ice on/across her naked buttocks until the ice has melted. Dry the spankee's buttocks if so desired and administer a good spanking to the spankee.

b) After the first spanking is completed, start over with more ice and repeat this until you're done.

IF-THEN – This scenario can be used with adults, particularly in Domestic Discipline relationships. The number of spankings, spanking duration, intensity, length, implement used and number of spankings the spankee gets are set up ahead of time for a wide range of infractions. Over spending on a credit card would have a clear and previously defined punishment, as would being late for work etc. Couples can spend a lot of quality horny-time determining what punishments the submissive member of the relationship would get for which infraction.

IMPULSE SPANKING – Unexpectedly administering a spanking without warning and perhaps for no particular reason.

INSUFFICIENT DISCIPLINE – When the submissive party thinks (to him/herself, or out-loud) that the dominant is not disciplining him/her adequately or is strong enough emotionally to administrate the discipline.

JUICY BUTT – A bottom that likely is great for spanking (or one that someone thinks would be great for spanking.)

KNEADING (aka *Petrissage*) - The palms of the hands and/or fingers work the buttock's muscle and fat tissue. Kneading a spankee's bare buttocks is also popular before, during, and/or after a spanking.

KNICKERS DOWN – An English saying meaning "panties down" in preparation for the spanking she so desperately needs.

LEATHER BUTT - A slang term for buttocks that are comparatively insensitive to spanking and do not mark easily. With enough spankings many buttocks become less sensitive.

LESBIAN SPANKING – When women play with each other sexually, and that includes spanking.

LESBIAN SPANKING STORIES – Erotic girl-girl spanking literature.

LIMIT – The point where the submissive party is unwilling to accept any spanking related additional intensity, duration and/or experience.

LINGERIE SPANKING – Spanking while the pretty lady is wearing lingerie.

KISS OF THE PADDLE – When a blow from a paddle on the butt leaves a significant mark.

LAP-WRIGGLING SPANKING – (a.k.a. *Good Old-fashion Lap-wriggling Spanking*) – Wiggling while over a lap getting spanked. (This is more of an English term.) This wiggling likely is because the spanking is particularly intense or the spankee's ability to take a spanking is not too developed.

LIGHT SPANKING – This can be applied to a clothed or bare bottom. It can be administered by hand or via the use of a spanking implement. It should not be particularly painful for most spankees.

LONG, HARD SPANKING – A lengthy and intense punishment spanking meant to change unacceptable behavior.

MAINTENANCE SPANKINGS – (*Preventative Maintenance Spankings*) - Spankings administered on a regular basis to keep the spankee on the straight and narrow. Punishment spankings are administered in addition to these.

MARATHON SPANKING – Lengthy spanking sessions that might be part of spanking contest or simply for a couple to establish their own personal best. In some marathon spanking sessions the couple can take a short break periodically.

MARKS – (*Spanking Marks*) – A good spanking with more than moderate intensity (depending on how sensitive the spankee's bottom is) can leave the bottom a lovely shade of red. It also can leave light contusions and more significant bruises. These bruises (aka "marks") could remain for days or longer or they can be gone in hours. A spankophile is proud of these marks hence the phrase "wears her (his) marks with pride".

MEMORY RECOVERY SPANKING – Spankings administered to hopefully help the spankee remember things he/she had forgotten. The hope is that he/she can remember that forgotten thing while being spanked or afterwards.

M/f SPANKING – Male spanking female.

MODERATE INTENSITY SPANKING – A spanking administered with only moderate intensity typically will give the bottom some or more redness. It shouldn't make the spankee cry or leave marks. This all depends on how sensitive the spankee's ass cheeks are.

MOTIVATIONAL SPANKING – This type of spanking scenario can help the spankee reach their goals. Perhaps the goal is good grades in college, or weight loss, or quitting smoking. Motivational spankings can work (but like anything in life is not guaranteed to work.)

(1) Before the spankee embarks on their endeavor he/she can be given the first motivational spanking, which is a serious spanking that really show him/her that it's better to stick with the program. His/her subconscious mind needs to be motivated also and a really good spanking might do just that.

(2) Should the spankee fail to reach previously established goals, he/she should be very soundly spanked and otherwise punished. Other punishments can include corner time, not being allowed to wear cloths (when in private,) Bed Arrest, orgasm denial and other forms of humiliation can also be incorporated. Perhaps you'd also like to invite all your BDSM/kinky friends over to give him/her a spanking.

MUSICAL SPANKING – Spanking to the beat of the music and/or for the length of the musical composition. (Ever spanked to "Bolero"?)

Another great thing about music is that it might cover up the sound of the spanks hitting the spankee's bottom and noises the spankee utters as his/her bottom is reddened.

NAKED SPANKING – The spankee, and optionally the spanker, are not wearing any cloths.

NSA SPANKING – (No Strings Attached Spanking) – Casual spanking where a special relationship is not necessary.

OLD FASHIONED BARE BOTTOM SPANKING – These are the standard spankings we grew up with. *Silent Spankings* and many if not all spankings when the spanker is tied down to spanking furniture, likely are not in this category. This term denotes a hard or harder than normal spanking.

OTK – (a.k.a. *OTK Spanking*) – Short for *Over The Knee*. This is one of the most popular spanking positions. Its benefits include that the spanking can start quickly versus having to tie the spankee up. Also the spankee's private parts and ass, with all its features, are in easy reach for the spanker's use (assuming the spankee allows that.)

PADDLE – A rigid spanking implement that typically is quite a bit longer than it is wide. The thickness of a paddle can vary. Paddles can increase the intensity of the spanking blows and make spanking a less tiring affair for the spankers. Paddles are usually made of wood but can be made of other hard materials such as acrylic.

PARTY SPANKING – Spanking that takes place at social gatherings. This includes *Spanking Games* and *Group Spankings*. Party Spanking is not the same as *Spanking Parties*.

PLAYFUL SPANKING – This can be when the spankee gets only light to moderate swats or a limited number of quick swats. Consensual playful spankings might be used to break the tension.

POUTING - To make a facial expression that indicates dissatisfaction; sulking. This might be done by the spankee prior to the spanking or when there is an indication that a spanking will take place in the future.

PRIVATE SPANKING - These spankings are given in an isolated private setting with invited company only.

PREVENTATIVE MAINTENANCE SPANKING – See *Maintenance Spanking*.

PROFESSIONAL SPANKING – When money or material goods are exchanged for one or more spankings. Spankings are given professionally by *Spanking Theraphists, FemDoms, Spanking Demonstrators* and others. It could also be the opposite where it's the spanking model that gets spanked in exchange for money or material goods. (This includes spanking pictures and spanking video models.) *Charity Spanking* is when people are spanked in exchange for others giving money to one or more charities for each good spank the spankee takes.

PUBLIC SPANKING – (This includes *Exhibition Spanking*) – Spankings given in a public or semi public non-group spanking environment. (Not recommended!)

PUNISHMENT AGREEMENT – A *Punishment Agreement* is an oral or written agreement that defines what punishments will be given for what offenses. See *Spanking Contract* and *BDSM Contract*.

PUNISHMENT FETISH – The idea of being punished, or even of being punished in a certain way (such as being spanked) in some way turns on the individual and could be a re-occurring fantasy.

PUNISHMENT ROOM – A room, or area of a room (often the basement, bedroom or the dominant's study) where most of the spankings take place.

PUNISHMENT SPANKING - (*Discipline Spanking*) – These spankings leave the spankee's bottom red and marked. These are hard spankings meant to change a wayward spankee's behavior. Typically the female spankee (and sometimes male) will cry from these. Also applied as part of the punishment could be corntime, bedroom time and other punishments. Perhaps the spankee will only be allowed to crawl for the rest of the day/night if going somewhere in the house, (obviously privacy is required.) Maybe one punishment spanking will not be enough, or even two! The subconscious mind needs to know what he or she did is no longer allowed!

PURIFICATION RITUAL SPANKING – This spanking category is more on the spiritual side. It can combine enemas, massage, prayer, meditation and/or bathing for spiritual arousal and/or renewal.

PUSSY SPANKING – The vagina is lightly spanked for stimulation and/or punishment.

QUICKIE SPANKING – When time is limited, but the spankee must have a spanking, he/she can be bent over the nearest applicable furniture or go over your lap for an immediate spanking. Often this is when the spankee is already dressed for an occasion. A quickie spanking needs to be given instantly, likely without any significant preparation, waiting time, discussion, or scolding.

REAL TEARS – This indicates that what's occurring is a good hard spanking! Sometimes during a spanking video shoot, the spankee, in-between takes, has a bit of water put by her eyes to mimic tears. No need to do that when the tears are real!

RED BOTTOM SPANKING - (a.k.a. *Red Ass Spanking*) – A good spanking should leave the spankee with some or more redness on his/her bottom. A bottom that is covered with redness would be from a true *Red Bottom Spanking* that the spankee can 'wear' with pride! The red bottom may be accompanied with marks (bruises).

RELIGIOUS SPANKING – Religious spanking has a very long history. Men and women's buttocks have been beaten for, and by, religious authorities in many past civilizations. Certain members of Christian clergy are recorded to have spanked (women in particular) back when it was easier for them to get away with it. Inquisitioners would beat men and women, often without mercy, as they considered them to be an affront to god.

A part of religious spanking history that may be of interest is how often women in the medieval and post medieval centuries, (often coupled women,) would request a spanking from the clergy (such as their minister or priest) as atonement for their sins or as confidential punishment for something isolated that they did. Often their husbands okayed it. Heck it was a lot better than going to hell right, at least that was what they thought.

Some church building basements had a separate section for these atonement sessions. This happened more often than people realize.

REWARD SPANKING – (1) When a spankophile just can't get enough spankings that you are actually able to reward her/him by giving a spanking. (2) A FemDom might consider all spankings she gives to her slaves to be a reward, or should be viewed as a reward. Punishment for bad behavior is typically more severe than a reward spanking.

ROMANCE SPANKING - This is for spanking couples involved in a romantic relationship. The spanking can be mixed with sexual stimulation and intercourse.

RULER – (Wooden Ruler) – Though often made of wood, it can be made of other substances. Some rulers are thicker than others and somewhat longer than one foot. The thick 1½ foot ruler is a dandy! The yardstick can be very useful for those long reaches, for instance when the naughty girl is sucking on a man's cock and he wants to spank her at the same time. (Watch out for those teeth!)

SAFE SPANKING – Don't spank too hard. Some spankees' butts are able to take more abuse than others, at least until the butt toughens up (assuming it does.) Also you want all parties to feel secure with the location and privacy of the place selected for the spanking.

SANDPAPER CHAIR – After the spankee is spanked, he or she sits naked on sandpaper. An alternative is to rub sandpaper on the spankee's well spanked bottom and/or run your fingernails over the spanked buttocks.

SCHOOLGIRL SPANKING – The naughty (adult) schoolgirl discipline fantasy is one of the most popular spanking fantasies. She is dressed in the pelted skirt and white dress shirt (perhaps also with a tie) and is constantly getting in trouble so she is constantly spanked! All female spanking enthusiasts (spankees) should have a schoolgirl outfit!

SELF-SPANKING – Spanking yourself.

SEXUAL DOMINATION – (Associated with *Sensual Domination*) - The dominant person controls and orchestrates the sexual relationship and sexual activity with the submissive person.

SERIOUS SPANKING – (1) Spanking enthusiasts that take the art of spanking seriously. (2) A hard or even severe spanking and typically is reserved for punishment.

SERVANT SPANKING – (Also see *Slave Spanking*) - Spanking of servants (though in past centuries and millennia they more often were slaves) occurred often. In those days masters and mistresses lorded over their servants with more power than they do today. If the lord (or mistress) of the house thought beating the servant would make good discipline (or simply enjoyed it), that was the servant's fate should she wish to continue working there, or often anywhere else as employment references were important.

The servant girl might be spanked for pleasure by the master of the house. She might be enjoyed in other ways too, though not as often from vaginal intercourse. Servant girls that ended up taking the role of concubines might be treated better and have less mundane work to do. Wives in those days were frigid move often than now. This might be because they were afraid to have too much sex with their husbands as it was so much easier to get pregnant back then thanks largely to a pronounced lack of birth control and the stricter demands of the prevailing religious forces that were staunchly against birth control. (Also women died during childbirth a lot more frequently back then.) A surprising number of wives simply considered the sex demands of their husbands to be too much and welcomed their use of a servant in that manner if it freed them from that arduous duty, (assuming he did not get her pregnant and kept his distance from her emotionally.)

The mistress of the house might order someone to be spanked (beaten) and perhaps do it herself. Husbands and male friends (or other servants) often were happy to do the beating for her, assuming it was a female getting spanked.

The person being beaten may or may not have the area being beaten, fully exposed (thus naked.)

SEVERE SPANKING - This type of spanking can cause much redness and/or severe bruising (marking), blistering or worse on the buttocks of most spankees. The spankee likely will find sitting a challenge for a certain amount of time. This needs to be done in a consensual manner and might not be legal.

SILENT SPANKING – (1) When the spankee is not allowed to utter any noise while being spanked. (2) Alternatives to spanking that quietly give the butt pain, such as the application of capsicum cream (but a very small amount) and the less effective Tiger Balm. Do not put it on the anus or sex organs.

SLAVE SPANKING – See *Servant Spanking*. (1) In the modern world of BDSM (*Bondage, Domination, Sadism and Masochism*) the submissive person is called a slave and is under the influence and/or control of the dominate party typically called the "Master" (if male) or "Mistress" if female. The submissive slave is dominated and spanked when the dominant feels it is necessary for discipline and/or pleasure. (2) (See *Servant Spanking* for more on this part of the definition.) Slaves in ancient times often were considered part of the family. They may have been expressly gotten for purposes of physical and sexual pleasure. They were spanked publically and privately in Roman and Greek locations at the whim of their owners. In the more modern slave ownership period including the Caribbean and in North America, black slave girls would also be used for sexual gratification when their owners wanted it. Also other male slaves might spank other slaves for various reasons, particularly when they were a supervisor.

SLIPPERING - Using a slipper as the spanking implement.

SOOTHING CREAM – (Cold Cream) - A cream applied to a well spanked bottom to limit the sensation of pain.

SOUND SPANKING – See *Hard Spanking*.

SPANKABLE – (Spankworthy) – The person is well suited to be spanked. They may appear to have an ass, due to its shape and/or appearance, that appears particularly well designed to be spanked. The mannerisms of the person should scream "spank me"! A professional spanking actress should have great "spankability".

SPANKED TO TEARS – When the spankee is spanked hard enough to cry real tears. Bad girl!

SPANKFEST – A synonym for "Spank Feast". This is a gathering, public or private, where spanking is one of the primary events (or at least is publicized to be.)

SPANKING ART - (Spanking Comics) – Spanking themed art.

SPANKING AGREEMENT - An oral or written agreement regarding spanking related activities. See *Spanking Contracts*.

SPANKING BEGINNERS – *Spanking Beginners* typically have little or no significant experience with giving a spanking and/or receiving a spanking.

It's important that the beginner's first spanking (or first few spankings) are as positive an experience as possible. Does the spankee want it to be a sexual experience also, if so then make sure sexual stimulation is accented. A bad experience now could turn this person off from spanking and another butt is lost to the spanking world :(

SPANKING BLOG – A (preferably) regularly updated online diary/web magazine that individuals and organizations keep regarding spanking pursuits.

SPANKING BONDAGE - When bondage is included with the spanking. Typically this means that the spankee is securely tied down and immobile for his/her spanking. Perhaps he/she is tied down to a piece of spanking furniture.

SPANKING CLUB – These associations provide a way to meet and/or otherwise intertwine with others in the spanking scene. They're sometimes called "Munches". Spanking clubs have grown quite a bit in number in recent years.

SPANKING CONTEST – When couples compete with spankings for a prize or prizes. The rules vary from contest to contest. Possibly included are:

A) Extra points for the spankee with the reddest butt
B) Extra points for the nicest looking marks
C) Points deducted for blistering or appearance of blood (typically then the spanking is over for them anyway)
D) Extra points for sexiest spankee's behavior while being spanked.
E) Points deducted for the spankee trying to block blows or get away
F) Points deducted for the spanker tiring too quickly
G) Extra points for the spankee with the sexist outfit and/or the outfit most conducive to making the spanking easier
H) Extra points for the spanker/spankee couple that is the most fun to listen to during the spanking

I) Extra points for how sexy and submissive the spankee is during and at the end of the spanking. She will have to beg for forgiveness, etc.

J) Extra points to the couple that uses the most spanking implements during the spanking

K) Extra points to the spankee's bottom that feels the best after being well spanked.

L) Extra points to the spankee that gets the most aroused

M) Extra points for the spankee with the most spanks during that time period.

Multiple spankings can be going on at the same time. Also see *Duel Spanking*.

SPANKING CONTRACT - It's a good idea for the participants to sit down and talk about their spanking scenarios, including under what circumstances the spanking will take place, how the spanking will be delivered, number of swats, instruments to be used, position of the person to be spanked, whether spanked with clothing on or bare bottom, etc. All participants then have an oral agreement on the terms, or have a signed written contract on the terms. This author sells a *Spanking Contract* through your ebookstore.

SPANKING CURRENCY - This is when spanks take the place of money, more specifically in place of your country's currency. How many spanks do you have in your spanking account? What are you going to buy with them? Or perhaps you are making a trade? Do you have a debt to pay off?

A common "spanking currency" scenario is paying off a debt. The spankee gets spanked in exchange for the debt.

SPANKING DANCE –The sub/slave does a sexy dance in front of her dominant and is spanked at various parts (times) of her dance. Perhaps it's after the end of each song, or if her dancing is not of an acceptable nature.

SPANKING DEMONSTRATION - When spanking partners demonstrate various aspects of spanking, including spanking implements and the best ways to spank.

SPANKING ENTHUSIAST – (Spankophile) - Someone who enjoys spanking, either receiving or giving. This includes activities related to spanking such as spanking media, building spanking furniture and spanking modeling.

SPANKING FANTASY – (Spanking Fantasies) – Mental images that run through one's head associated with spanking. A great many people have these.

SPANKING FOR COUPLES – Adult spanking activities that couples involve themselves in.

SPANKING FURNITURE – These apparatuses are used to place and secure one or more spankees. These include whipping benches, the spanking horse, the birching horse and the spanking bench. The spankee may or may not be tied down to it. The spankee often will find him or herself in the kneeling position or bent-over position. There should be easy access to their buttocks and often spanking furniture make the buttocks the most elevated portion of the spankee's body. Also being able to take and/or play with the spankee sexually while on and/or tied to spanking furniture is of pronounced importance.

SPANKING GAMES – (1) Online interactive games where the players determine who gets spanked and the intensity of the spankings. A spanking game may let the player interactively spank one or more characters. (2) Physical games such as Strip Poker that calls for one or more participants being spanked at various intervals. This type of spanking game typically has a way of determining who the spankee is and who the spanker is.

SPANKING HOST – The host or hostess at spanking social events and online and real-life spanking clubs.

SPANKING IMPLEMENTS – These physical devices are used to aid and enhance the delivery of the spanking blows. Examples include paddles, straps, slappers, floggers, rods, switches, canes, spanksticks, crops, the tawse and whips. Not everybody agrees but some people feel this category also includes restraint aids such as handcuffs and rope.

SPANKING LIFESTYLE – The world of spanking is innately intertwined into the lives of the spanker and/or spankee.

SPANKING MAGAZINE – Content from these wonderful periodicals now are often also online.

SPANKING MASSAGES – Combining full or partial body massages with spankings. The massaging may be the primary activity or vice versa.

SPANKING MASTURBATION – (1) Masturbating during and/or after a spanking and masturbating on those days afterwards while your bottom is still sore from the spanking. (2) Being spanked for masturbating.

SPANKING ORGASM – An orgasm that is obtained while one is being spanked, or while their buttock is still smarting from having been spanked in hours or days since the spanking.

SPANKING PARTY – Spanking parties might be in a home, a hotels or resort and are a gatherings specifically set up to accommodate spanking. Often there tends to be a significantly higher percentage of males at these events than females.

SPANKING POSITIONS – The bodily location of spanker and spankee just prior to, during and just after the spanking.

SPANKING PRACTIONER – See *Spanking Enthusiast*.

SPANKING REMINDER – This often is a short but relatively intense spanking session to make sure the spankee remembers to be obedient and/or is reminded as to what kind of punishment awaits her should she do something wrong.

SPANKING ROLEPLAY - There are many role-play scenarios that can include spanking. Naughty nurse, submissive maid, naughty schoolgirl, misbehaving cheerleader and warden/prisoner role playing is popular with male dominants and female submissives.

Spanking Roleplaying can require acting and props but it always includes a generous helpings of spankings.

SPANKING SERIES – A sequence and/or collection of spankings and/or spanking characters, stories, videos and/or pictures, which have certain characteristics in common.

SPANKING SESSION – Most associated with visits to FemDoms and Spanking Therapists. These are often "visits" that have a purpose but it still can be just a girlfriend and boyfriend meeting for fun.

SPANKING STICK – These look a lot like manmade canes.

SPANKING STORIES – (*Spanking Novels, Spanking Novellas, Spanking Series, Corporal Punishment Fiction, Flagellation Erotica, Romantic Spanking Stories*) – These are literature adventures involving spanking. These go back to the 1700s and may or may not involve sexual activities. The Marquis de Sade is among the most famous of these authors. In the past these tended to be clandestine publications that were sold secretly.

SPANKING THERAPIST – A person that administers *Spanking Therapy*.

SPANKING THERAPY – This aims to help spankees improve themselves. Perhaps he/she needs more motivation or just the tension release of a good spanking. The spanking is conducted by a professional. The spankee's needs are assessed and addressed in a controlled, nurturing environment (assuming nurturing is what the spankee wants.)

SPANKING VIDEOS – Spanking videos have proliferated with the Internet. As is obvious, these videos show spankees getting spanked and often dominated in other ways.

SPANKING WITH **ANAL STIMULATION** – (1) Directly stimulating the anus while giving a spanking (which can include aiming the blows at the anus and/or to make the blows include the anus.) It can occur before a spanking, and/or in between spankings, and/or after a spanking. This might involve inserting a butt plug (inflatable or otherwise), finger(s), anal vibrator, a dildo, or rectal thermometer into the anus. It might include carefully spanking a dildo that's already put into the anus to make it move up and down in the anus as blows are applied to it and the buttocks. (2) Actually spanking the anus with a narrow spanking instrument. (Spanking related enemas are a separate subject, see *Enema Spanking*.

Anal stimulation doesn't necessarily include anal intercourse.

SPANKING THE MONKEY – Male masturbation.

SPANKOPHILE – – (*aka Spanking Enthusiast*) - Someone who enjoys spanking, either receiving or giving. Their interest could also include spanking implements, discussing spanking, spanking media, building spanking furniture and spanking modeling.

SPENCER SPANKING PLAN – A well known domestic discipline spanking contract that originated in the 1930s.

STING AND THUD - Thinner spanking instruments such as switches release their energy closer to the skin and thus 'sting' more. Thicker spanking instruments such as paddles release their energy down further in the buttocks making more of a "thud" sensation.

STRAP – (aka *Leather Strap*) – A spanking instrument of various sizes that can be deliciously effective. It's often made of leather and thus is pliable.

STRESS RELIEF SPANKING – (*Tension Relief Spanking*) - The aim of these spankings are to eliminate frustration and guilt and cleanse oneself mentally. At the conclusion of these spankings relaxation and comfort can be had by the spankee.

STRUGGLING – When the spankee fails to hold his/herself adequately in place for/during and after their spanking.

SUBMISSIVE SPANKING – When the spankee wants to feel dominated as part of the spanking, over and above the domination involved with him/her getting spanked.

SUBMIT AND OBEY – A Dom/sub lifestyle outlook where the submissive submits and obeys his/her Dominant.

SWITCH SPANKING – Where the spanker and spankee take turns spanking each other.

SWITCHING – (Associated with Birching) – A switch is a flexible thin branch (rod) from one or more trees. (A collection of thin branches can be tied together to also be used as a spanking implement.) A switch is applied with force to the buttocks of the spankee. The switch like the cane can hurt more than many other spanking implements due to its thinner surface area so caution is advised. Also see *Caning*.

TENDER – The tendency for the buttocks to become sensitive to the touch after a good spanking.

TENSION RELIEF SPANKING – See *Stress Relief Spanking*.

THRASHING – This term is more popular in England and denotes a hard spanking/beating often with one or more implements.

TICKLE SPANKING – (1) Tickling the buttocks and then spanking it (an act that can be repeated.) (2) Tickling various parts of a person's body such as their belly and the bottoms of their feet, and also spanking that person's buttocks, alternatively or simultaneously.

TIT WHIPPING – Spanking the breasts of a woman using one or more implements. This can only be done consensually and with caution.

TRADITIONAL SPANKING – This denotes standard methods of spanking. No unusual methods of buttocal pain infliction, such as *Silent Spanking*, would be included in this category.

TOP UP SPANKING – These are given regularly, even every few days, even in addition to any other spankings the spankee has received. These spankings are for bad behavior that the spankee got away with during that time period (say week) and for bad behavior she might be tempted to do in the following week. See *Maintenance Spanking*.

TOUCH-YOUR-TOES – When in a standing position the spankee may be ordered to reach down and touch as close to their toes (perhaps their knees) as possible so their buttocks can tighten and stick out thus becoming an easier target to spank.

TOUGHEN-UP SPANKING – These spankings (and spankings in general) if given with regularity, can dull nerve endings in the buttocks as well as toughen tissues in the buttocks. The spankee might evolve into having a "leather butt" which is a butt that can take a disproportionately hard spanking.

WAKE-UP SPANKING – This well helps to wake up sleepy beauty and typically works much better than an alarm clock.

WARM-UP SPANKING - This is a light spanking, often by hand and perhaps on a clothed bottom, before the "real" and more intense spanking begins. Its purpose is to prepare the butt for the coming onslaught.

WEARS HER (HIS) MARKS WITH PRIDE – (*Spanking Marks*) – A good spanking with more than moderate intensity (depending on how sensitive the spankee's bottom is) can leave the bottom a lovely shade of red. It also can leave light contusions and more significant bruises. These bruises (aka "marks") could remain for days or longer or they can be gone in hours. A spankophile is proud of these marks hence the phrase "wears her (his) marks with pride".

WEIGHT-LOSS SPANKING – If the spankee needs motivation to lose weight, spanking can be of use. The spankee can be spanked whenever weight loss goals are not reached and/or can have the more desirable reward of a pleasurable spanking when the goals are met. Perhaps the spankee should be given a hard spanking just before the diet is to begin to remind him/her what's in store if transgressions occur.

WELL-SPANKED BUTT – A buttocks that has the tell-tale signs of having gotten a good spanking.

WET SPANKING – For this the spankee's butt is made wet. It can also be when the spankee wears something wet that covers her bottom and is spanked over that. This can enhance the pain coefficient.

WHEEL BARROW SPANKING POSITION – The spanker sits up and the spankee lays her hands on the floor directly in front of the spanker. The spankee spreads her legs and brings her ass and legs up over the sitting spanker's lap. Her legs are positioned on each side of his upper torso. Her pussy and anus are spread wide open next to his midsection. Her ass cheeks are on his lap, her spread open pussy lips are facing him.

WHEEL BARROW SPANKING – When the entire spanking is administered with the spankee in the wheel barrow spanking position (see previous definition.)

WHUPPIN – Slang for whipping.

WOODEN SPOON – This kitchen implement can also double as a spanking implement. Bad girl!

The End

Book #5 - Bare Bottom Spanking – The Las Vegas
Spanking Adventure

By Jim Rollins

Bare Bottom Spanking –
The Las Vegas Spanking Adventure

I want to tell you about an incredible spanking adventure I treated myself to in 2009.

My company temporarily transferred me to Las Vegas, a city in the midst of a terrible recession.

I had hoped to meet some kinky ladies to play with, in particular to spank on their bare bottoms, but when I talked to them in casinos and bars, too often they ended up being sex workers (prostitutes) versus eligible single ladies so finally I decided to just go with it.

I put aside $1,000 and planned on spending it all on spanking call girls on their bare bottoms, (and any sex that came along with it.)

I put a few ads online explaining that she would give me a massage, then I could play with her as I wished and she would get spanked good and hard on her bare bottom. Her butt would be red and marked and any girls that couldn't handle it need not apply. I even asked for pictures of their previously well spanked butts as reference. I also told them to expect their hands to be tied together as this spanking would hurt.

I would pay each sex worker $200 cash. Happily I was gifted with many inquiries from the ads. Allow me the pleasure of telling you more about them.

1. September 17th, Wendy - This shapely brunette was "kinky", 5'4" and 135 pounds according to her online advertisement. As she wouldn't verify online or on the phone how much of a spanking she could take, I met her at a casino bar and we talked for a while. She sure was cute. Her top was cut so low her breasts threatened to fall out when she walked. She was dressed as a sex toy and I sure hoped this was going to work out as my little man downstairs was real interested in her.

A neat thing about meeting a sex worker at a bar in preparation for playtime is that you got to socialize with a (hopefully) fine looking lady, though not for long if things didn't work out. This time however it did.

I showed her pictures of well spanked girl's bare bottoms and told her that is what she should expect. She asked for more money (this would happen often with the girls.) I politely refused. She finally agreed and insisted she could handle it.

We went back to my place. She freshened up in the bathroom, came out and stripped. (I had the $200 on top of the TV.) Her butt was a bit loose but very spankable. Her tits were firm and lovely (she later said they were recently enlarged.)

I was on the couch. She knelt down in front of me and said she was ready to do whatever I wanted. As I was also naked I thought what the heck and told her to suck on my cock. Hmmmm that was a good move too! She sucked like a pro and I was hard in a jiffy, however I was here to start my spankfest as I just had to have this monster spanking memory to look back on when I was old and gray.

As tough as it was to pull myself away from her surprisingly strong mouth, I did. I told her to get my bag of spanking implements and put it on my right side. With her eyes wide open she said something like "wow you're prepared." I ordered her to once again to kneel in front of me and I tied her hands together.

Well the time had come. I told her to lie over my lap with her head on the left.

Spending a little time massaging the delicate bare bottom that was about to get roasted seemed only fair, as well as teasing her pussy with the vibrator. She clearly enjoyed both, particularly the later.

I put the vibrator down and pulled out a black 12 inch long leather slapper, resting it on her butt, making her moan in anticipation. "You know what to expect young lady. Now stay in place or it will only get worse."

"Yes Sir" she meekly said, fidgeting.

I lifted the slapper up and *Whack! Whack! Whack! Whack!* I spanked her lovely bare bottom with precision, this was going to be a long night for it and I wanted to make every inch of it red. Yes 'redness' was tonight's key word!

WHACK! WHACK! Smack! Smack! SMACK! She started moaning and breathing deeply. "Ow that hurts!"

"Well it's supposed to hurt young lady." I reminded her. SMACK! SMACK!

She tensed as she wondered what was now to come, then she began yelping regularly as she felt the slapper repeatedly come down hard across the curve of her bare bottom. She regained her breathing as I temporarily rested the slapper on her butt. She then felt the slapper lift off her posterior and she heard it whistle through the air as it came down again on her vulnerable ass, time and time again. She was now crying out with each strike and reeling from the barrage of blows. I then stopped and exchanged the slapper for a paddle to continue her spanking. The paddle would make her squeal and kick her feet. The spanking continued.

After what felt like an eternity to her I stopped and she flinched while I rubbed her reddening butt. "This looks great" I said impressed as her bare bottom was reddening nicely. "Imagine what your ass is going to look like when were done....Lucky girl!"

SMACK! SMACK! SMACK! She yelled as she felt the paddle come down on her ass again and again, "Please sir just use your hand" she begged. No way I thought, that was not part of the bargain. *WHACK!* That felt harder she thought and indeed she was right, I had exchanged paddles, this was a bigger one. Well at least it wasn't a cane she thought. She hated the cane. But still, knowing that it wasn't the cane didn't lessen the pain of the spanking. She yelled each time it struck. I counted fifty new blows on her hot, red, marked bare bottom before it stopped. What a sight she was, crying and kicking her feet like a naughty schoolgirl.

I stopped to admire the view. This was indeed a great memory in the making.

"Please stop, oh please sir!" she begged.

"Are you going to be a good girl?" I asked firmly. "Yes sir I promise" she responded submissively. I wanted to let her go right then but I wanted my money's worth of bare bottom spanking. Yes one more volley on her red, marked bottom would do the trick.

Slap! Spank! BAM! Slap! Crack! Spank! Bam! I spanked down her upper legs but stopped fearing that the redness on her legs would show out in the public as she was wearing such a short dress. Instead I went back to paddling her upper and outer bare bottom as those regions weren't as red. SMACK! SMACK! SMACK! The crying she had started a while back was making her even more sexy. This was really a great way to start my Las Vegas spanking memory.

Well the spanking finally ended and I let her down to kneel in front of me. Her hands were still tied so she couldn't rub her red well spanked bare bottom that well even though she desperately wanted to. I would do that for her instead. It was hot and a lot of fun to rub. I was holding her close as I bent down to rub her red, marked bare bottom and rake it with my fingernails. She was still snifling.

"Suck on my cock young lady and drink down all my cum. If even a drop is lost we start your spanking all over again." "Oh god no" she begged and eagerly started sucking on my cock with her tied hands massaging my balls. Soon I would cum and true to her word she drank down every drop of my cum.

She would call me again periodically asking if I wanted another session but she insisted on more money so it never happened.

2. September 24ᵗʰ, Jennifer - Jennifer was actually the first to answer one of my online ads but after I responded back to her, I didn't hear from her for 9 days. She had insisted that she was a spankophile and "could suck every drop of cum out of me." Oh course she wanted more money but eventually agreed to the $200 as money was so tight in the recession.

Since we had talked on the phone (and I even had her smack her own bottom with a ruler many times while on the phone to prove she meant business,) I decided to just let her come over. Later that night the door bell rang and even though I was only wearing a bathrobe, I let her in. She took the money and put it in the purse. We talked a bit and I gave her a drink to loosen her up. She then pulled out a leather strap from her bag and asked me to only use that on her. I agreed.

Jennifer had long red hair and nice tits with cute little nips. Her best feature though was her round, tight ass. It looked like it was begging to be spanked. She told me how she loved to feel the sting of the blows and the jiggling of her bare bottom which she could feel all the way up her spine. She said a good hard spanking impacts all her sexual points, her nipples get hard like little pencil erasers, her pussy juice starts dripping down her inner thighs, and her asshole quivers. A big cock, spankings and my red ass cheeks that come along with it, really gets me off she said in the sexist way.

Well that description had come out of the blue and sure left my cock hard. I got the impression on the phone that she was into being spanked but this was even more than I expected. I removed my bathrobe and presented her with my newly hardened cock. Her eyes had been transfixed with my midsection since she walked in and seeing my big, hard cock made her quickly strip. I particularly liked seeing her see-thru pink panties. She knelt down in front of me and began sucking on my little man with a vengeance.

I reached down and played with her tits. My cock generously provided her with copious amount of ooze, which she lapped up as she softly moaned. I then reached over her back and played with her cute tight ass. She must work out as it was so firm.

Oh oh, I was about to cum so I lifted her head off my cock, put her hands together on my lap and tied them together as she shuddered with anticipation. She was really turned on now, her heart was beating fast partly out of nervousness and partly out of lust.

"Spread your legs as far as you can and keep your eyes on my cock" I told her as she was kneeling in front of me, soaking wet. I reached down to her pussy and spent some quality time playing with her clit. It took very little to make her cum, however it wasn't for near as long as she would have preferred.

I then told her to lie over my lap and Las Vegas spanking number 2 began.

Smack! Smack! Smack! I used my entire hand on her ass cheeks making it land repeatedly right on the fleshiest part...SMACK! SMACK! SMACK!

I was in a blissful state of ecstasy after giving her 40 hard blows. I pulled her ass cheeks apart and slide 2 fingers in and around her pussy just to tease her. I know she needed to cum again. I know she wanted to squirt all over my lap right then and there to relieve the tension in her aching pussy. But no way would I allow that.

But now back to the business at hand. I renewed my vigor and spanked her bare bottom harder. Jennifer went from moaning loudly to crying out as the blows came down hard and heavy. *WHAP! WHAP! WHAP! SMACK! SMACK!* Her ass cheeks had reddened quickly. One never knows who's ass will reddened the fastest. "Your ass reddens quickly, I like that" I said still spanking. She just moaned loudly, no doubt wishing I'd take a vibrator to her pussy.

SMACK! SMACK! SMACK! The leg kicking had gone into full swing now. It was fun to watch. It didn't slow down my spanking though. BAM! BAM! "Oh please stop" she half heartedly cried out. I knew how that goes thought, she didn't want it to end at all.

Hmmm the lower ass cheeks weren't as red as the middle so paddling there became the latest order of business. *WHACK! WHACK! WHACK!*

"Please fuck me, oh god please fuck me" she begged as I continued in my spanking quest. *BAM! BAM! BAM!*

"Beg for my cock in your pussy, beg for it slut!" I bellowed still spanking her red ass hard. *SMACK! SMACK! SMACK! SMACK! SMACK!*

"Please, fuck me, fuck my red, beaten ass!"

Well fucking her well spanked butt was an unexpected request but man was I ever ready for that.

"I will keep spanking your bare bottom until I don't have any energy left, or I can stop and fuck you right now in your ass, which would you prefer young lady?" "Oh god yes fuck me in my ass now please" she pleaded.

And that was that, another spanking in the books. I let her off my lap with her hands still tied together. I told her to get on the bed. I quickly got some petroleum jelly, a small towel and a condom.

She was on her elbows and knees with her swollen pussy lips facing me. I could see pussy juice dripping off of her. I got on the bed behind her and lubed her ass generously with my finger. I then wiped my finger off, put the condom onto my already hard cock and looked down at her red ass with delight wondering what she was thinking.

Jennifer had felt the prodding and lubing of her asshole stop, only now it was replaced by the feeling of my cock pressing into her little ass opening. She knew it would hurt a little but she loved to be fucked in the ass, even if it hurts at first. I slowly stuck it in, pressing past her sphincter and thrusting all the way inside. Her asshole stretched to accommodate my cock.

"Mmmmmmmmmm!" She let out a moan as I pressed into her. She was ready to cum. She wanted me so badly to touch her pussy, or for her to even just to rub it with her bound hands, then, unable to wait any longer, using her bound hands, she played with her clit, screaming out as she came.

With a big thrust my dick was inside her ass. I started thrusting slowly but worked my way to thrusting into her fast and hard. She let go and came with abandon.

Well that was definitely a memorable spanking experience but like all good things it came to an end. Jennifer spent the night, we had breakfast out the next morning and she went her way, though would call periodically.

3. September 30th, Tiffany – Tiffany knew Wendy, the first sex worker I spanked. Wendy told her of my spanking quest and she was anxious to join in the fun, and make some money!

We talked on the phone but I didn't hear from her for a few days. Suddenly one night I get a call and she is wondering if she could come over right then and there for her spanking. I said sure! When she got there however she first asked if she could take a shower. Perhaps that was to clean off the smell of the other johns. I said sure. She was in there around 20 minutes. Spanking memory number 3 was about to begin.

I told her not to bother getting dressed after she showered. I had undressed myself and laid all the sex toys and implements out, (as well as the $200.)

Through the closed door of the bathroom I said that she was a bad girl for taking too long with her shower and she was going to get a good spanking.

She came out, naked and looking very excited. She looked at me real seductive like and said "Have I been a bad girl? Are you going to spank me?"

"Yes young lady you have been a bad girl and you're going to get a good spanking."

Tiffany was curvy. She weighed about 150 pounds and had C-cup breasts. They hung down a bit but were still nice. She clearly was very turned on.

"You've needed a good spanking for sometime haven't you young lady?" "Yes sir" she said, her eyes fixed on my hardening cock.

"I'm going to bend you over this chair and I'll spank your ass good and hard for being a naughty girl."

All she could do was hang her head and stare at the floor. Her pussy was so wet that she had pussy juice running down her thighs.

"Answer me slut." I commanded.

"Yes..." She stammered now as she was confused as to how she got so turned by all this so fast.

"Yes what slut?"

"Yes sir." She replied quickly.

Her clit was throbbing, so she started to rub it. "Don't you dare touch yourself without my permission young lady" I quickly said. "Please may I touch myself sir" she begged.

Without answering I went over and grabbed her hands pulling her over the back of the chair. I tied each hand to different chair legs, then stopped and looked at my handiwork.

She looked scared like maybe she was concerned I was a weirdo and she had gotten herself in too deep.

"Don't worry Tiffany, you are not in any danger but you're going to get one heck of a spanking!"

That made her feel better and she said "Yes sir I'm a naughty girl. I need to be spanked. I want to be spanked. Spank my bare ass Sir."

"Say it again, and say it louder."

"Yes sir, I'm a naughty girl, I need to be spanked, I want to be spanked. Spank my bare ass Sir" she said trembling as she stared at the carpet.

As she was submitting so readily to me I decided to lube up her anus, maybe I'll take her in it after her bare bottom spanking. I could see that her nipples were rock hard. She looked up at me and saw that I was staring right at them. As I lubed her ass with a dildo she looked back and watched, moaning with pleasure. She also saw that my cock was already hard.

It was time. I then walked behind her and started to spank that lovely bare bottom. *WHACK! WHACK! WHACK! WHACK! WHACK!* Red hand prints appeared on her ass as she let out sexy yelps with each blow. SMACK! SMACK! SMACK! SMACK! SMACK! "Hmm, nice ass" I said and kept spanking her. *"Oww, ohhhhhh, ahhhhh"* was her reply. Still it was clear that she was loving it as she began pushing her ass out to meet my hand.

My hand flew up and down, crashing down again and again on her firm bare bottom. I gave her around 60 hard swats when I noticed sweat was forming on my brow. My arm was also starting to tire. No problem, I have another arm and I went to her other side so I could use my left arm instead. BAM! BAM! BAM! BAM! *"Ohhhh please owwwwwww"* was all she could say.

"Let's see how wet you are slut" I took a break and reached down between her ass cheeks, feeling for her pussy. I pushed one, then two fingers deep in her pussy. She lifted her head and moaned with pleasure. "Wow are you ever a wet little naughty slut that likes being spanked and is hungry for some cock. I bet you want it up the ass right now, don't you?

"Yes." she stammered, her face burning with shame and excitement. Stealthily I grabbed a paddle.

"Yes what?" I said punctuating the question with the paddle. WHACK! *"Owwwwwwww"*

"<u>YES SIR</u>!" She replied. The sting of the spanking had spread to her pussy; the sharp blows of the paddle were leaving an impression. Oh how that paddle burned her ass and yet she still pushed her ass back for more. She wanted more, she wanted to be paddled like the naughty slut she was. She also wanted desperately for his big cock to be in her mouth, her pussy, her ass.

"Yes sir what?" He asked again, spanking her more and hard with the paddle. *WHACK! WHACK! WHACK!*

"*Yes sir I want your cock in my ass.*" She cried.

Well I had been spanking her for around 15 minutes and her ass was beet red. Clearly this was a good spanking but I longed to use the paddle more on her, and that's what I did.

WHAP! WHAP! WHAP! SMACK! The paddling went on and on bringing a big smile to my face. She was crying and begging for it to stop. After another quick 20 more swats, the spanking was over.

I reached down and tied each of her feet to their respective feet of the chair. She squirmed some but I was too strong and she wasn't in a good position to do much. She now had her hands and legs tied down to the chair. I then came around her front and stuck my cock in her eager mouth. She sucked on it for all she was worth. "Suck hard young lady or I start your spanking all over again."

I stayed there getting my cock sucked hard, though it was a tough thing for her to do with her hands tied and her upper torso hanging over the chair, still she knew better not to do a good job sucking.

As nice as her sucking was it had come time to take her on the other end. I pulled out of her mouth, dried my cock off and put on a condom. I went to her backside and quickly rammed my cock deep in her soaking wet pussy, fucking her for all I was worth.

"*Oh god yes!*" She cried out as he filled her pussy with his hard cock. She began pumped my cock as much as the ropes would allow.

I reached under her and fingered her clit knowing it would send her over the edge. "*Yes! Yes! Yes!*" *she cried.*

It was great to feel her pussy contract around my cock as she came again and again.

But she still had a nicely lubed ass left to fuck and I wasn't going to let that opportunity pass me by. I pulled out of her pussy (to her objection) and entered her ass, soon cumming hard with a shout.

Well that was another great spanking and fucking session. Dang Las Vegas can be a fun town.

4. October 7th, Cindy - Cindy was another working girl that knew one of the girls I had already played with. I talked to her several times as initially I got the impression she was not sure if she wanted to be spanked. Actually I had given up on her when she called and insisted we do it. I wasn't convinced and actually I was the one that refused. Then one night, out of nowhere, Wendy (who I had already spanked) called and said she was bringing Cindy over and that I could do whatever I wanted with her, for the $200 of course. (I would later find out that Cindy owed Wendy money and needed cash fast which is why I was supposed to pay Wendy and not her.)

Wendy also wanted to know how well Cindy preformed as Cindy was in trouble with some important people and had to perform well or leave town. She said that people were glad she was going to get punished and urged me to redden her ass but good. Wow, suddenly I had a lot of power over this naughty young lady.

After she arrived I immediately ordered her to stand in the corner. I informed her that tonight was all about punishing her and should she refuse anything people would hear about it, people she'd prefer didn't. With a lump in her throat she submissively said "Yes Sir."

I sat on a chair and inspected my evening's entertainment. "Remove your dress slave" I barked "and don't you dare look at my eyes for the rest of the evening."

She quickly removed her dress and put it in the closet, going back to the corner when she was done.

"Pull your panties down to your knees." I ordered. Slowly, almost fearfully, she pulled her sheer black panties down. As Cindy pulled her panties down, she exposed her lovely rounded ass cheeks. Wow what a spankable ass. "Take three steps back" I said. She did. "Now remove your panties and bend over and put your hands on the wall." She did.

"Spread your legs slave." She did with some hesitation. "Spread them further and don't even consider disobeying me." She spread her legs a couple of feet further. I was now able to see her lovely brown asshole and her pussy lips. I walked over for a closer look. She was shaved all the way from her pussy to her ass, only a few days of stubble was present at most and she had nice healthy pussy lips.

I could feel the blood surge into my cock. I took off my underwear and was now naked.

"Please don't hurt me sir. I'll be a good girl" she begged submissively.

I ignored her. "Go lay over the big chair with legs spread and with your hands spread your cheeks slave, I want to see more of that beautiful ass and pussy."

She obeyed and using her hands spread her ass cheeks.

"Young lady, you are beautiful. You have a fantastic pussy and ass. Stand up and take off your bra, I want to see your tits." I told her.

"What are you going to do to me sir?" She said looking down. I must say I was impressed, she was in a bad position but was remained composed, however she had not yet removed her bra.

"You are going to be my sex toy this evening young lady and I am going to punish you at will as well as enjoy you in any way I wish." I told her. "If you young lady are in anyway uncooperative, I will tell those that want to know."

"Please sir, I'll do whatever you want, I promise" she begged.

Her hands went behind her back and she unbuckled her bra. She let it down and I got the full view of her big, beautiful tits. Her areola were brown and about the size of a half dollar coin. I watched as her nipples became erect from the cool night air.

"I expect nothing but obedience from you from now on. Do you understand that slave" I said to her.

"Yes." she replied.

"Excuse me" I roared.

"Yes, sir" she quickly said.

"Now that we have an understanding, come lay across my lap. It's time for your first spanking of the evening and then we get on to other things...NOW!"

She hurried to me and hesitated for only a moment as she went to lay down on my lap as I sat on the couch.

"Put your pussy directly over my legs." I told her. Now her nice ass was in easy reach.

"Thirty to each ass cheek should be a good warm up" I told her as my hand reached back, ready to strike.

"Oh please, noooooooooooooo" she cried.

I chose her right ass cheek, the one closest to me, for the first volley, and using my hand I spanked her hard... *WHACK! WHACK! WHACK! BAM! BAM!*

Her ass cheeks jiggled as my palm went from cheek to cheek and she cried out with each blow. I watched with great satisfaction as her cheeks quickly got red. *SMACK! SLAP! SMACK! SLAP! SPANK!*

She struggled, moaned and cried out but didn't try to get up. "Would you like me to stop Cindy? You know what will happen if I do."

She whimpered, "No sir, please don't stop."

I started to smell pussy juice. I pulled her ass cheeks open and could see her pussy was getting lubricated, hmmm looks like she was getting turned on quite a bit.

WHAP! SPANK! BAM! WHACK! SPANK!

It was great to watch her lying across my lap, her bare bottom already red. The smell of her wet pussy was a nice touch.

"Are you ready for the paddle young lady?" I asked sarcastically.

"Oh no" she cried, "Please no sir"

"You have such a spankable bare bottom. It will be tough for me to stop spanking you." *SPANK! WHAP! SPANK!*

"Spread your cheeks for me slave" I ordered her as I ran my fingers over her now red bare bottom.

She obediently reached back with trembling hands and spread her burning red ass cheeks. Reaching onto the small table beside me, I got some lubricant.

"Keep your cheeks spread. Should they stop being spread at anytime without permission, you will be in so much trouble young lady" I firmly told her. I heard a quiet sob as she dug her nails into her ass cheeks to keep them spread open wide. Her brown, wrinkled anus was a very inviting sight.

I lubricated my middle finger. Once it was well lubricated, I put my right hand between her legs and my left hand on her back. I leaned forward and gently caressed each of her lovely pussy lips.

My slave for the evening gasped, but did not move. I took exceptional delight in watching her anus flex uncontrollably as I caressed and teased her labia. Her body was reacting on its own to my playful touches. I could see the lips of her pussy becoming plumper from the anticipated invasion. I pushed my index finger between her lips and felt the hard little button of her clit. I heard her gasp.

As I continued to massage her clit, I let my lubricated middle finger rest against her anus and the other fingers against the inside of her right ass cheek. I started to flick my finger harder and faster across her clitoris and she started to uncontrollably pant.

"You have 15 seconds to start cumming from this slave but if you move from your position I will very, very severely punish you." I told her as my right index finger now rubbed against her clit harder and harder.

Cindy tensed and then began to orgasm. I was glad to see her cum. I was still going to beat her plenty more but I wanted her to love being forced to obey me. I planned on this being a very long evening for both of us.

Cindy cried out as she came, her ass cheeks and thighs straining to remain open, I could see the muscles in her back twitch as she came.

"Stay in position slave or I'll make your tits as red as your ass." I said sternly.

I took my index finger away from her clit and watched her shudder. Her pussy lips were completely open.

I started to massage around her anus with my middle finger. Once her asshole was slick with lubricant, I began to massage her anus with my middle finger, gently probing the edges and the entrance to her ass, but not penetrating.

"Please, not my ass" she begged.

"What?" I said.

"Please, not my ass, Sir." She said.

"Now you're just being funny" I said with a smirk. Wow how nice it was having a sex slave for the evening.

I said nothing but continued to massage her anus. Cindy didn't squirm but periodically I could feel her anus tense and relax. Soon though the sphincter muscles fully relaxed.

Without notice I penetrated her ass with my big middle finger. I curved my finger up and could feel her tailbone. My slave girl gasped once again.

I continued to explore her rectum with my middle finger. I'm not sure if it was fear or sexual ecstasy, or a combination of both but she was moaning hard with pleasure.

Now, I changed direction and pressed down toward her pussy, searching for her G-spot.

She let out a guttural scream as I found her G-spot and I used my thumb to play with her clit as I also probed her G-Spot through her anus. I made her cum again.

Cindy sighed as I removed my fingers, but I wasn't done with her ass yet. I took out a butt plug and inserted it, making her cringe.

"Young lady, if this butt plug comes out without my permission, I will whip your tits with my belt"

"Oh god, please no sir" she said suddenly scared.

I then took a paddle and once again the spanking onslaught continued. *SPANK! SPANK! SPANK! SPANK! SPANK!* She cried out but was careful to keep the butt plug in. *WHAP! BAM! SMACK! SMACK!* I now started spanking fast and hard, the hardest and fastest of the night.

"I dare you to move away slave. I just dare you." That stopped her fighting and her bare bottom would stay in place for the rest of the onslaught. *"Owwww, Ahhhhh, pleaseee sir."* Her ass which had lost some of its redness while I played with her, got it all back. It was once again the way a punished girl's ass should look, red and marked. I particularly enjoyed making the paddle land on the butt plug that was mostly buried in her ass.

I put the paddle down and once again fucked her ass with the butt plug, enjoying her moans. "Soon it will be my cock in there, not just a butt plug."

I told her to get up, which she did slowly, as the experience was draining her physically.

I sat on the edge of the bed and she knelt in front of me so she could suck on my cock. After 10 minutes of that I could take no more without cumming and told her to get on the bed on her hands and knees.

Well you can guess what happened next, I took her in her pussy and then her ass, thus concluding another great Las Vegas spanking memory.

5. October 15th, Tracy – Tracy answer my online ad. We chatted online but I thought she was too bitchy so I wrote her that I wasn't interested in her. Two days later she writes back and apologizes for giving the wrong impression. She also wrote that I could take it out on her butt. Well that's all I needed to hear. Just to play it safe I arranged for us to meet at a casino salad bar for dinner.

Unfortunately I once again sensed that she wasn't really into getting a good spanking but just curious, and wanted the money. My experience was that for the hardcore spanking I wanted to do, girls that are just curious wouldn't get through it. So I later excused myself.

6. October 24^h, Ginny – Well I had heard a former girlfriend that I had lived with had moved to Vegas some years back but I had misspelled her last name so I couldn't find her. One morning while I was fresh from sleep I suddenly remembered her last name's spelling. Hopefully she hadn't re-married and was using that same last name. As luck would have it she hadn't and we made contact.

We talked some on the phone and decided to meet for dinner. When I finally saw her I was concerned. She had lost 10-15 pounds and her breasts were Bs instead of the Cs I lived with. Bs are good though. She still had that schoolgirl look and worn a low cut dress. She looked tired and maybe not well bathed. However she seemed like the same nice person that unfortunately had fallen on hard times.

She explained how she had recently lost her job, car and roommate. Her credit was shot from less than frugal spending.

I asked her why she stopped writing me and she said from shame. She hadn't taken care of business as well as she should have in life.

"When you and I were together, thanks to your rules, accountability and discipline, I had direction in life which was so good for me. I went from living with my ex-husband who wouldn't hesitate to beat my ass with his belt to you who also kept me in line the same way."

We had lived together for several years and as I listened I could tell where it was going.

"You set limits for me, and when I exceeded those limits you punished me. I never realized how good for me that was."

I would spank Ginny often. Spanking was for foreplay and harder spankings were for discipline. I always had remembered all the hot discipline sessions we had. She was right, those sessions did her a world of good and I always wondered how things would be for her when she got transferred to the east coast by her company.

"You showed me that you cared and loved me by soundly spanking my bare bottom." She looked up at me with questioning eyes, "are you still a spanker?"

"With all my heart and soul" I answered knowing how badly she longed for a good, hard spanking.

She sat silently for several seconds took a deep breath and said. "Tom, I think what I need is for you to give me a good hard bare bottom spanking, would you please do that?"

I was not surprised by the request as I knew her well enough, and knew she needed it badly. "I would be happy to and I know that's just what you need."

Dinner was over soon and I drove us back to my place. I informed her that she would do exactly what I told her to do for the rest of the evening, which she agreed to. I had her take a shower and brought out her old schoolgirl outfit for her to wear. Amazingly I still had it. She thought that was great. She put it on though it was a bit loose.

I told her to bring a cushion over and kneel down in front of me and that he could no longer speak unless she's spoken to. The evening's discipline would now commence.

Her white schoolgirl dress shirt was buttoned up and she was wearing the bra she came here with.

She looked up at me longingly which was sweet but she would not be allowed to look up without permission. I reminded her of that and she apologized. I cut her slack as it had been so long that we last had a discipline session.

I then proceeded to chew her out for her undisciplined behavior. It made her cry. She repeated that the only way for her to get her act together is with discipline and she can't be allowed to get away with acting the way she had in the past.

I removed her white schoolgirl dress shirt and her bra and played with her tits as I scolded her. Her nipples were still sensitive and she moaned with my touch.

Wow, it was so nice to see a pretty girl that so desperately wanted a good long hard bare bottom spanking. Actually I could hardly believe my good fortune! But back to Ginny.

"Tonight young lady will be a night you will always remember because this begins our new journey together, a journey that will see you be all you can be." She felt very moved and while keeping her eyes down thanked me. I leaned down and gave her a long kiss which made her moan. While I was kissing her I reached down with both hands and massaged her asscheeks. They were warm from the shower but soon would be downright hot.

I pulled her hands up to my lap and tied them together. There was fear and anticipation in her eyes.

I then looked down at her and said "the time has come young lady, get over my lap." She looked scared but obeyed by laying over my lap with her head on my left.

I was prepared too. Next to me on the right side were a number of paddles, straps and sex toys.

"You should feel free to cry young lady as this is going to be as hard and as long a bare bottom spanking as I've ever given you." With that I brought a paddle down with moderate force. She exhaled and clinched her creeks.

"Sir" she said, "I haven't been spanked in a long time." "Well then we'll make up for lost time" I said reassuringly.

Ginny swallowed feeling a lump in the back of her throat. She felt strange but she liked that he cared and wanted to help her deal with her lack of discipline. She knew he knew how to change her habits and disposition. Then suddenly she was thinking of something else. The spanking had begun and now she was thinking of only one thing, the pain on her bare bottom.

SPANK! SPANK! SPANK! SPANK! SPANK!

Oh that's what a spanking feels like she thought, now I remember. Wow that's hurts but it was making her feel warm all over. *Finally a spanking!* She clasped a couch cushion and moaned progressively louder and louder. SPANK! SPANK! SPANK!

"During the spanking, when you're really sorry about the way things have been lately, I want you to apologize for letting it happen." "Yes sir" she whimpered. SPANK! SPANK! SPANK! SPANK! SPANK!

"Owwwwww, ohhhhhhh, I'm sorry sir." "Good girl but you're going to need a lot more of a bare bottom spanking for things to start to sink in."

Her moans were now cries as I spanked a lot harder and faster with the paddle. I would not hold back. I had carte blanche to beat sense into this young lady and that was what I was going to do. Tonight she learns her lesson, Tomorrow she has trouble sitting.

Periodically Ginny would relax her feet but quickly cross them again as the pain of the blows reminded her why she was here. She wanted to put her hands on her bare bottom to try and rub some of the burning sensation away, but they were tied in front of her. She tried gritting her teeth as he beat her tender behind. She started to pull her ass away but stopped when I threatened to start the spanking all over from the beginning, as well as spank her just as hard for the next 5 night in a row. Wow, five nights in a row, that would be a sexual sadist's dream come true, though I doubt if her butt could take it.

SPANK! WHAP! SPANK! WHACK! WHACK!
"Ohhhhhhh, owwwww, I'm sorry sir, please stop."

I wasn't even thinking about stopping this spanking. The thought had not even crossed my mind. I would however take a rest at some point and have her stand in the corner in preparation for round two.

She was crying now, here cries were punctuated with each swat. Yes this bad girl was really learning her lesson.

"Oh god I'll be good I promise" she wailed kicking her feet. I was expecting the foot kicking so I stopped spanking long enough to put my right foot over her lower thighs to keep those in place.

I was impressed at how she still retained her ability to take a hard bare bottom spanking. Her submissive nature remained intact in many ways. I enjoyed the nostalgia of looking at an ex's well spanked bare bottom, one I hadn't seen in years.

SPANK! SPANK! SPANK! SPANK! SPANK! Then she tried to get up. "Even think about trying to get up again and all you get is the cane until I'm too tired to swing it." Hearing that made her scream. What a horrid thought. She would work harder at keeping in place. *Whap, Whap, Smack, Spank, Bam, Spank!* "Are you going to get your life in order young lady because I can do this to you every night" I secretly wished I could do this to her every night! *"Yessss sirrr. Owwwww."*

Her ass was mostly red and nicely marked. She was crying with real tears. Significant however was that I was tiring. The spanking would stop for now and she would spend sometime in the corner. I released my leg from over her legs. "Get up and kneel in front of me." She fell over my lap and quickly knelt in front of me trying so hard to rub her tender bare bottom but could barely reach them with her tied hands. As she sniffled I reached down and massaged and kneaded her well spanked cheeks. "Remember you have been ordered not to speak unless spoken to" I reminded her.

As her bottom was already so well spanked, maybe a second one would not be advisable after all; well the second one can be lighter.

Playing with her ass calmed her down some, now it was time to play with her breasts. I lifted myself up some and made myself at home with her breasts and their now firm nipples. Her sniffling was slowing and being replaced with moans of pleasure. "Hands on my legs" I ordered and she eagerly put her hands high on my legs.

"Now suck on my cock."

Her eyes were on it the whole time and she eagerly began sucking.

Unfortunately I was so turned on that I couldn't hold my orgasm back and soon filled her mouth with my cum. Fortunately she still remembered the importance of sucking down every drop of a man's cum.

Having orgasmed, I lost a good deal of my sexually sadist desires for the night. I let her go with just that spanking (though it was a nasty one.) I took her in her pussy and ass later that night and she moved in with me two weeks later. I'm happy to say that she is doing great and so am I.

My wonderful Las Vegas spanking adventure had a great ending. Wow about yours?

The End

Book #6 - Hera's Kinky Playtime in Ancient Greece

By Selene Thaleia

Copyright (C) 2013

Hera's Kinky Playtime in Ancient Greece

Chapter One

Hello I'm Hera, a young woman and slave in Corinth. I don't know what year it is but Persia has already invaded us once.

My owner is a military commander and shield maker. (Our shields are called "hoplons" or "aspis".) He is very demanding and strict. He controls my life in almost every way. Master took me prisoner when his small army of 200-400 men (called a "tagma") conquered my village. Both my mother and father had passed away several years ago, my mother from an illness and my father in battle. My aunt had taken care of me. I was 20 at the time and I, like whoever else they wanted, became a slave to the conquering warriors from Corinth. It is the standard way of doing things in my time. My aunt always warned me that if Corinth ever wanted to conquer us, as I was so pretty, I would certainly be taken as a slave. She was right.

Master is a firm believer of discipline and that includes keeping his slave well disciplined. He has a big collection of paddles, slappers, straps, whips and more. It's my job to keep them organized and in order. I pleasure my master many times a week. I'm also available to any of his friends if he wishes.

Master spanks me on average about twice a day. It's something he genuinely loves to do. Usually master always gives me a spanking before bedtime. That spanking is among my favorite as it helps make me sleepy. If a friend comes over that's interested he'll let him spank me also if they want. I don't think he thinks I can be spanked enough. I am not allowed to wear any cloths at home unless we are expecting company or if it's cold. Master also has a cage that I get put in, often in preparation for playtime or if he's angry with me. When Master is aroused I have to particularly be careful as he'll punish me for the smallest of things.

Master's friend Master Adrēstos came over for a visit yesterday and as usual I was tied up naked on the half table, spanked and taken. The half table is several feet long with stirrups so my legs are kept securely straight up in the air. My arms and lower belly are strapped to the table. My ample breasts thus are securely in place should they be the focus of attention, as they often are. On the half table my pussy (called "kolpos") and anus are right on the edge of the table so they can be played with and taken with ease. When I'm being spanked on my tits or ass I usually will be required to cum ("orgasmos") at some point, which is no problem for me. Yesterday while taking me in my ass (rarely am I ever taken in my pussy,) Master Adrēstos finally let me cum and wow was that ever a great orgasm.

Typically in the morning I wake up and fix Master breakfast if he wants it. He may call me into his room to pleasure him if he is in the mood. Before he puts on his clothes, master gives me a good over the knee spanking before he goes to work. He says it helps get his blood pumping and be more ready for the day. Those morning spankings can really wake me up fast. It's usually always with a paddle. Master doesn't usually spank me with his hand anymore, he used to when he first got me. As Master is paddling me in the morning, he will tell me what he wants me to do that day, assuming there is something he has on his mind.

I have to admit that today was different as Master started the day very angry with me. I was supposed to go to our neighbor and get the olive oil he promised us but once again I forgot. After I admitted forgetting to get the olive oil, he lectured me about being forgetful. He hates it when I'm forgetful; unfortunately it's something I have a problem with.

I knew I was in a lot of trouble. I could see he was winding up to spank me really hard. I apologized of course but that rarely does any good. He ordered me to put the klismos (chair) in the middle of his room and get the large black wooden paddle. He ordered me to bend over the chair so my hands were on the chair seat and my butt was the highest thing on me. I looked back at him as he came over, careful not to look at his eyes of course. What I saw made me cringe. He looked really mad. He was scolding me as he ordered me to count out the swats. He started by tapping my butt many times with the black leather strap. It was a something he made especially to spank me with. It's falling apart but still hurts a lot. He started right in on my butt with it. *Slap...slap...slap...SMACK, SMACK, BAM, BAM, SMACK, SMACK...* Sure I'm required to hold still but it's not easy when he gets in a mood like this. I began moaning after the 8th spank or so then gave progressively louder yelps after the 15th. Usually though I can take a very hard spanking. Maybe my butt's toughen up a bunch over the years.

Master kept scolding me about forgetfulness and laziness. He's had trouble with me about this before. Smack, smack...smack, BAM, BAM, BAM. My butt cheeks were bouncing around from the blows and getting redder and redder. Since Master was pressed for time I think he spanked harder and faster. After the 60th or so spank I was begging him to stop. *"Ow master, pleaseee I'mmm soorrry."* I was flinching and moving my outstretched butt which is something that unfortunately made his madder. He grabbed me and held me in place as he really laid it on my ass. I knew it was getting red by then. SMACK, SMACK, BAM, BAM, SMACK, SMACK. Finally he stopped but instead went to get a small strap. "Move away or block even a single blow and you'll spend the next two days in the cage slave." "Yes master". I meekly said holding on to the seat with all my might. BAM, BAM, BAM, BAM. *"ow, ah, pleasseee, no moore master."* BAM, BAM, SMACK, SMACK, BAM, slap…slap, slap. "What is my favorite color for your ass slave" master howled? ""Red sir," I sheepishly muttered. "I'm now going to check your pussy and god help you if you're not soaking wet". Master's rule was that I had no more than 30 seconds into a spanking to have a wet pussy. This spanking had lasted a lot longer than that already. He must have not woken up completely because he's usually checking me sooner than that. Master is always looking for a reason to punish me and that would be one of them. I felt his fingers enter my pussy and feel their way around inside of me, he teased my clit and I started to cum immediately but I'm a well trained slave and know better than to cum without permission. *"Master, please may I cum, please, please."* Of course he wouldn't let me cum then and his fingers withdrew, soaking wet. Master rubbed my hot red ass for a bit but I knew the only thing that would stop this spanking would be his not wanting to be too late for work. That's one of the great things about our morning spankings. Master doesn't have a lot of time to complete them. "Stand up slave" he ordered and I pushed myself up from the chair rubbing my sore butt. Master caught me rubbing myself. "Hands behind your back slave." Master then took the heavy wooden ruler in hand and sat on the chair I was just bent over. "Lay over my lap now." I quickly complied, my open palms on the carpet and my toes were also on the carpet. I would have to stay this way or the spanking would never stop. That was the rule. Master rubbed the heavy wooden ruler over my ass. "I love how red your ass gets from a good spanking" he said. "Thank you master." I mumbled. The truth was that by rubbing the ruler over my well spanked ass like that felt good, but that sensation would abruptly change. BAM!! Wow no warm up but hard spanks right from the start. BAM, BAM...SMACK, SMACK, BAM, slap...slap, smoosh, slap, bam, BAM. I was crying now. *"No please Master, I'll be good, I swear."* BAM, SMACK, SMACK, BAM, slap. Tears were willowing up in my eyes . ""Ow master, I'm sorry, I won't dooo it again, I swearr." Now master was spanking me in rapid succession. He really like spanking that way. The side and the top of the right cheek was getting most of the attention for 2 or 3 minutes then it was the left cheek's turn. After 30 or so really hard swats on each cheek, his spanking tempo slowed and his spanking intensity slowed. The end of this spanking was near. "There" Master finally stopped the deluge and looked down at his slave's reddening ass proudly. "A job well done. Get up. You may rub yourself." I stood up and furiously rubbed my butt. This was definitely a harder spanking for a morning spanking than usual; little did I know how much more was to come.

Master sent me to stand in the corner. I still was rubbing my ass but the sniffling had stopped. Master liked to hear me cry after getting a good spanking. He came over to me on his way out of the bedroom. He pulled my hands away from my butt and started rubbing my hot, red butt cheeks. Suddenly it dawned on me what could happen, I couldn't believe I had just thought of it. "I'm going to ask some folks to come over while I'm gone and have them also punish you. You will give them sex also if they want. You will remain naked until I tell you differently." "Yes Master" I gulped.

Several times before Master has had friends come over to the house to punish me. I have also had to go to their homes and get punished at their convenience. Sometimes master has parties and slaves like me would entertain the masters and mistresses. Those that allowed it would let their slaves be played with by the others. Typically all the participating slaves, male and female would go one at a time to each master and mistress in the room and ask how they can serve them. Usually we would be spanked and have our pussies and tits played with. Some would require that we cum from it. We also would give hand jobs and blowjobs and eat their womanhood if they wanted it, and of course it would be our responsibility to clean up after the men came. The lucky masters and mistresses though got to do a lot more with us later.

After a female slave had gone around the room serving the masters and some of their wives, she would be tied down on her back to a table, her anus on its edge, (nobody could take us in our pussies) and the masters and mistresses would take turns taking and/or playing with her. I remember one night, while tied down, helpless and vulnerable, my ass was taken 9 times. My asshole would feel so hot afterwards. I suspect it was all the friction. Often I would be sore for several days from this. Of course I had to cum for everybody that took me which wasn't as easy later in the night but I didn't want to be punished. I should note that the masters weren't only taking me but also taking the other female slaves so they wouldn't spend as much time in me as they would normally.

Anyway, as Master was leaving, he said that he would be back for lunch to punish me again and he would also send Master Coenus over this morning to punish me as well. Then he told me the terrible news.

"I am going to take care of your laziness once and for all slave." Oh oh, this didn't sound good. "Today you will get spanked 9 more times. And I mean good spankings. If that doesn't do the trick it will be repeated 2 or 3 times a week from now on. You know I'll have no problem finding people to spank you and if I have the time that won't even be necessary."

My mouth dropped open. "But Master it will hurt so much." "Good" was his reply. Master Coenus should be here to spank you anytime now." With that he hung up. I was stunned. I tried to think back to the most spankings I've had in a day and if it was a day that included one of those sex parties, I'd say 15 but the spankings I got at a sex party were usually short and often not that hard. Oh my gosh. Suddenly I wasn't horny at all but concerned.

Clearly this was going to be a long day. Happily Master released me from the corner as he walked out the front door and I now had some time to collect my thoughts.

Chapter Two

My butt heals fast, probably because it's been spanked so much. Its redness goes away surprisingly fast and frankly Master doesn't like that. He'd prefer watching me walk around the house naked with a well spanked, red, marked butt. Bruises show up on my butt but they too go away surprisingly fast. The fact is I would need all those physical characteristics to get through this incredibly spank-filled day.

I put the paddles, straps and other spanking implements away in the closet where they hang or lay in draws. I made master's bed. The house had 3 rooms. One room was master's bedroom, one room was a main room, where I also slept and another room was a playroom where master and his friends did whatever they wished to me and others. That room also had the cage I got put in sometimes, as well as furniture that master had made to tie me down to. The kitchen as well as the bathroom were outside.

Master had ordered me to be naked so I didn't have to decide what to wear. I went out to the kitchen and proceeded to clean it up.

I laid down on my bed recalling the already busy morning. Just then Master Coenus walked in "Your owner asked me to come by and give you a good spanking. I hear you were forgetful again." "Yes sir" I muttered. "Very well, go fetch my favorite paddle, the brown and gold one." "Yes sir."

The brown and gold paddle was a gift to my master from a friend. It's about 2 feet long and maybe a third of an inch thick. It has holes in it and a black leather handle. It's nasty but I have a very tough butt.

I went to the play room where the cage is and friends of master's spank and play with me the most. Master Coenus had already gotten out of his cloths. "Crawl to me slave". I quickly got down on all 4s and crawled to him, giving him the paddle. "Kneel in front of me slave, hands on my legs." My mouth was now only a couple of feet from his cock. Unexpectedly I felt a tremendous urge to suck on it. My horniness had returned. "Suck" he ordered. Master Coenus was pretty predictable. I would suck on his cock for a while as he spanked me with the long paddle. Fortunately I am well trained and won't clamp my teeth down on his manhood as he spanked. The intensity of his spanking at the moment was not that hard. He was after all being sucked and didn't want to tempt fate. I do have teeth. I knew from experience that he would soon stop spanking and play with my breasts as I sucked on his cock, invariably ordering me to cum. Oh Zeus I can't wait! I lost track of how many spanks I was getting. I was however ready to cum but knew better than to try to ask. "Faster slave". My head bobbed up and down faster on his cock as I feverishly played with his balls. Master had always taught me to play with a man's balls while I was sucking on his cock. Holding a thin stick, he would watch me as I sucked on a cock to see if I would dare disobey him in that regard. (As I noted earlier, he is very strict.) If he thought I was not playing hard enough with a man's balls he would say "head up" and I would lift my head off of his cock and he would beat my ass to everyone's delight.

Then it happened, Master Coenus reached down and commenced playing with my breasts. He was always good at it. I stopped sucking momentarily and begged "please sir may I cum?" He said yes and I nearly saw stars. I had to keep sucking hard though or he'd stop playing with my breasts and immediately start my beating. I shuttered some and hesitated momentarily but caught myself and kept sucking as hard as I could. I thought I did quite an impressive job to be honest. I made gurgling noise as I sucked and came. My tits kept being played with, it was great. After about 10 minutes of heaven I was ordered over his lap as he sat on the couch. Oh that's right, the spanking, that's mainly what he's here for. Well at least I was recharged after that orgasm. Besides my butt was already broken in for the day, how bad could it be?

The other thing I wanted to mention is that Master Coenus was a very sensual master and liked his slave playmates to cum a lot. He is kind enough to start the paddling easy and worked his way up to the hard stuff. "I hear you are being lazy and forgetful again and your owner wants that to end." He was spanking now as he spoke. "Yes sir" I managed to say. He was spanking faster and harder now. *BAM, BAM, SMACK, slap, slap, smoosh, slap, bam, BAM.* He was spanking harder than usual and man it hurt. "I had a slave that was lazy and this is just what I gave her. You cannot spank a lazy forgetful slave too much." BAM, SMACK, SMACK, BAM, slap BAM, SMACK, SMACK. "Yes sir" I was now trying so hard to hold back tears. *"ow, oh, pleassse no moorre, oow, oh, ow"* I mumbled. He then spoke "Your master insisted on me spanking you good and hard and that slave is what I'm going to do." He was now spanking real hard and in rapid machine gun-like fashion. That was it. The dam broke and I started crying. *"I won't be lazy sir I prooomise."* I started kicking my legs some but I knew better than to move my butt away. Darn Master Coenus was strong too. Suddenly he stopped. I couldn't believe it. "Give me you right hand". I gave it to him and he pulled it across the small of my back, now he had made me more immobile. "Beg for the spanking to continue." *"Please sir, spank me more."* Like that was an easy thing for me to say. "You can do better than that" he roared. *"Oh please sir beat my ass until I have learned my lesson and will be a very good girl."* Well I got my wish and the paddling continued. SMACK, BAM, slap, BAM, SMACK, SMACK. "Oww" was that me that just said that. Wow it was. "Legs spread" he ordered and I quickly spread my legs. He spanked in the areas down by the pussy, the areas that were still white, areas that my Master hadn't even gotten to in his haste. Oh gosh, I have another spanking from Master coming up at lunchtime, and this one isn't even over yet. SMACK, BAM, slap, slap, BAM, SMACK, SMACK, slap. My ass cheeks were bouncing back and forth. Then suddenly he ordered me to cum. I went from *"please stop, ow, ow, oh"* to making guttural sounds and not feeling the paddle at all. "I'm cummingggg" I screamed as I rubbed his legs with my pussy as hard as I could, still the spanking went on, slap, BAM, SMACK, SMACK, SMACK, SMACK. He was spanking very evenly from one cheek to the next, upper cheek then lower cheek and some on the upper legs but I continued to cum as ordered; then suddenly the spanking stopped. His hand went down to my pussy and finger fucked me. I arched my back and came even harder for him. I don't know where he found all that energy but his fingers were going in and out of me so fast. Finally he stopped. He then ordered me off his lap to continue sucking on his cock. I hesitated at first as my orgasm was still going on even though nothing was touching my pussy or clitoris (which is a Greek word.) I worked my way to his cock. "Suck" he ordered and my mouth went back to work.

I rubbed my ass cheeks with one hand and played with his balls with the other. Once again my cheeks were hot and red. I was dying to look at them but knew better than to stop sucking. I was tasting a lot of Master Coenus's ooze and knew what was coming. He came with a shout and filled my mouth with his cum. He held my head in place on his cock. *"Faster slave"* he ordered and forced my head deeper onto his cock. I drank down all his cum. For many minutes I knelt there making sure to drink down all off Master Coenus's cum. Finally he got up and got dressed as we talked. "I hear you're getting 10 spankings today and that could be repeated soon". "Yes sir." "Well maybe I'll stop by again this week to give you another one." "Yes sir;" like I had a choice.

With his clothes back on, Master Coenus left. My red butt still stung but I came so hard during the spanking that I'd have to consider that spanking a breeze. I wish master would let me cum more often when he spanked me but my Master is strict, demanding and controlling. Most of the orgasms I got from Master were when he took me in my ass, something he enjoyed doing very much. (As I said earlier, few of us female slaves got taken in our pussies.)

Sometimes master would allow me to lay in bed with him. Master is very proud of his property. His hands would wander when lying in bed with his slave girl. Sometimes his fingertips caressed, other times his nails scraped as he explored his slave's body. My nipples would get a lot of attention. When master tired of such torment, perhaps he'd tie my hands together. He would then take his time choosing what toys to use on me next. Perhaps earlier I didn't move fast enough or I made too much noise, waking him from his nap. Or maybe he's just in the mood to paddle my butt. My ass is his property to do what he wishes with after all. He would bend me over his knee and run his nails over my already well-spanked ass. His spanking starts slow and gained momentum: slap, slap, slap, SMACK, SMACK, SMACK. Once my ass is a lovely shade of red he'll send me to fetch his paddles, whips and rope. My bound hands are hooked to the ceiling high above my head, so I have to stretch up on my tiptoes. Then he works my body over with his paddles and whips, gentle taps punctuated with hard smacks. When he's done beating me, he lets me down. With my bound hands in front of me I am lead to his bed. He strips and lays down with his cock on the edge of the bed. I am then ordered to pleasure him. He enjoys watching me wiggle into a position that allows me to put my mouth to good use.

With my well-spanked naked ass now sticking up and out, if someone else walks by I will inevitably get played with. Master likes to watch mistress' play with me also and will invite them over to watch them do just that, often while I am sucking on his cock.

Master's lunch break started soon. I had to have lunch ready soon. He would spank me first, then eat. That way he had cooled off a bit before heading back to his job as a military leader and shield builder. It was always the same. He would sit on the chair where Master Coenus spanked me and then proceed to redden my butt there. I got all the implements he might want and put them on the table in front of where he would spank me. As he'll be in a hurry, it's doubtful he'll tie my hands together, even though he loves doing that before spanking me. As the sun got higher in the sky I made a plate of food for him, had something to eat myself and went and knelt by the chair in anticipation of my next spanking.

I was not there for long when he walked in and immediately sat in front of me on the chair. "Over my lap slave" he ordered and I crawled over his lap as I had done so many times before. "Your ass is still warm, nice. Now which of these shall I use?" Master first picked up a black leather slapper but put it down instead opting for a wide paddle. He rubbed my butt tenderly with his hands for a while, then with the paddle. "I see that between my spanking earlier and Master Coenus's spanking we're leaving our mark on your lovely ass. Perhaps after this day and night is done, you will have learned your lesson." "Yes master" I said.

Well the rubbing was fun while it lasted but then master started spanking in earnest. *SMACK...BAM, slap, BAM, BAM...BAM, slap, slap, slap.* I started squirming. "Hold still slave or you'll spend the next 3 days in the cage except to work, provide pleasure and be punished." Gee, that didn't sound like fun. I quickly gained my composure and largely stayed put. SMACK, SMACK, slap, slap, BAM, SMACK, SMACK, SMACK, SMACK... BAM, slap. My butt by now was tender enough for me to really feel the swats. *"Ow, ow, no please, ow, aw, aw, stop please, oh."* "I like that" Master said as he started spanking me harder. "Oh please no, ow." I grabbed once again the chair leg and held onto it with all my might. Fortunately my butt began acclimating to the blows and the pain tapered off some. Then master started with the irregular blows. I hate those. He'd rub my butt with the paddle then quickly raise it and bring it down on me, many times in rapid succession. *"Now let's see how fast I can give you 50"*. I didn't just hear 50 did I? SMACK, BAM, slap, BAM, slap, slap, BAM, SMACK. I was squirming as the blows really hurt. I tried to stay in place as much as possible. I raised and lowered my butt some from the pain. RAT, TAT, TAT, BAM, BAM, SMACK, BAM. *"Stop pleasssssse Master, I'll be gooooodd."* 29, 30, 31, 32, he counted out. I started kicking my feet some but caught myself and held back as much as I could. I cried out as he started the 40s. He was now spanking with all his might. *"Ow, no master, stop, oww, ow."* Abruptly master pushed me off his lap and dropped the paddle. I rubbed my scorching bottom. "Kiss my foot." I crawled over to master and kissed his left foot. "Lick it slave". I lathered it up with my tongue, then he pulled his foot away and bent over to inspect his work as I held my naked ass up in the air. "Not bad for a quickie. Tonight your tits get it also and it will be an all night affair. I'll give you all the spankings left to make 10 for the day. Now bring me my lunch" I quickly went into the kitchen and got his lunch. I then went back to being on my hands and knees. "You're going to have more visitors this afternoon. You'll take their punishment and serve them." "Who will be punishing me master?" "Master Mentes and Master Ponteus. Master Mentes should be here anytime. I need to go. Now go stand in the corner and wait for Master Mentes." "Yes master." I stopped rubbing my butt and walked over to the corner putting my nose against where both walls meet. I heard the front door close as master left with his lunch.

My butt was sore, three good spankings in this short of a period was the real thing. I turned my head hard to see how red my butt was. It was red okay and marked.

Master Mentes was a good friend of my Master and they have shared slaves before. I knew what a visit from Master Mentes meant, a tit whipping. Master Mentes loved to play with and beat tits. I've never seen anyone quite like him when it comes to that.

He has a tit fetish I think. On the other hand he sure knows how to make them feel good. I hope that today will be one of those times.

Chapter Three

Sure enough I didn't have to wait long. Master had left the door open and soon Master Mentes walked in. "Hello little one, your master requested my assistance in punishing you and I was oh so eager to be of service. Aren't you grateful?" "Yes sir" What was I going to say. "I haven't whipped those lovely tits of yours in a while have I?" "No sir." "Frankly I've missed them. I see you're undressed, good."

Master Mentes was quite good looking. "Come kneel in front of me slave." I took my nose away from the corner and walked over to him. He was sitting on the chair where I had recently gotten spanked. "Kneel". I knelt in front of him with my hands behind my head. He caressed and played with my tits. He had always really liked them. "Up high on your knees slave" he ordered. My breasts were now at his mouth level and he began sucking away on them. I begged to cum but he ignored me, as if he never even heard it. He pulled both nipples into his mouth and sucked on them at the same time. My knees buckled from the pleasure. I don't think it was an orgasm but I continued begging for permission to cum, no such luck.

Master Mentes then released my tits and pulled me towards him by the back of my head for a kiss. He had done this before but I had forgotten about it. He then had me remove his clothing. He then ordered me to suck on his cock.

As I've told you before, my orders are that when I suck on a cock, I am to stick my butt up and out so it can be enjoyed and otherwise used by others. By using long implements my ass can now also be beaten by the person I'm pleasuring. I hadn't seen it when I had originally come over but next to him, Master Mentes had put his short whip. "Suck harder slave" I heard him say as he rested the whip on my back. I sucked hard. At least I'm not going to get spanked hard if I'm sucking on his cock.

Master Mentes really took care of himself. I could tell by how good his ozze tasted. I love good tasting ozze and I lapped it up eagerly. Suddenly he began whipping my upturned butt. *FLOP, FLACK, SMACK, CRACK...CRACK, BAM...FLOP, SMACK*. The whip kept landing mostly on my butt but he also whipped my back. He wasn't beating me particularly hard, besides I didn't care because I loved sucking on his cock and the beating was just getting me hornier.

Suddenly it stopped. "Head up slave." I forced myself to stop sucking and took my head away from that lovely cock. I kept my eyes on it hoping that being away from it would be just a temporary thing, but it was not to be. "Your owner tells me your forgetfulness has returned and he wants it to end.' "Yes sir." "Clearly then you need quite a bit of discipline for such a thing. We're going to start with a spanking and then a tit whipping. You know how I love to whip those gorgeous tits of yours." "Yes sir." "Give me your hands." I clapped my hands together on his lap and he tied them securely together. He then motioned me to lay over his lap which I did. He began rubbing my already tender butt. "Legs spread". I spread my legs about 2 feet wide. He then stuck 2 fingers up my pussy. Wow did they ever easily slide in. "Wow, you are one wet little slave girl. Very good. But no you're not cumming yet."

Master Mentes started my spanking with his hand. He went right to work too, *SMACK, SMACK, BAM, BAM, slap, slap, BAM, SMACK, SMACK, BAM, slap.* I lost count as to how many spanks. I had also forgotten how much Master Mentes liked to spank with his hand. Now he was spanking hard, smiling down on me as I squirmed and moaned. "I don't accept forgetfulness in a slave so why should your owner? "I understand sir" was all I could muster. *BAM, BAM, CRACK, CRACK, slap, slap, BAM, SMACK, SMACK.* My ass was already tender from the day's abuse so I was feeling this more than usual. I kicked my legs some. Master Mentes was really laying it on fast and furious. Then suddenly I found myself on the verge of cumming. I knew Master Mentes wouldn't let me cum so why ask. I continued to yelp, moan and squirm. I thought I might cry when suddenly I started cumming, even though I didn't mean to. I tried hard not to move my pelvis in a manner that would give away that I was cumming without permission but suddenly Master Mentes's scolding and spanks meant a lot less. Then Master Mentes stopped using his hand, reached for a strap made of pig skin and continued the deluge on my ass, rubbing it periodically to admire his work. I had a nice controlled orgasm as he scolded and spanked me. *SMACK, BAM...BAM, slap, slap, BAM, SMACK..SMACK, SMACK, slap.* I turned back to look at my ass and it was red. "Eyes forward" he scowled giving me 5 really hard strokes to punctuate it. The spanking now was really hurting and as I had lost concentration, I also lost my orgasm, now all I felt was pain. *"Ow, noo sir, stop, oow, ow."* I pounded the floor in pain. He had never spanked me so hard. "Hold your ass still slave." I hadn't realized it but I had lifted my butt up some to avoid the spanks. Wow, that was a bad idea. He went back to work on my ass and upper legs, this time with a medium size rubber paddle. *"Ow, ooh, ooh, pleassee sir, I'llll be good."* Dozens of spanks later I was crying hard. I can take a really hard spanking but all this attention to my ass was really getting to me. Then suddenly it stopped.

"Kneel" was the order and I eagerly knelt in front of him as I rubbed my butt cheeks. "I see we have tears here" he said looking into my eyes. "Good. I believe the message is getting through to you." "Yes sir" I moaned while rubbing my naked, sore bottom. "Now it's time to give those lovely tits of yours the same kind of attention." Oh great, but at least my butt would get a rest for a change.

I had been trained to easily cum from breast stimulation. I am so proud of my breasts. They give me and others so much pleasure. They can take quite a beating too. Master Mentes specialized in tit torture so I suspected my tits would be red soon.

As I knelt in front of him, Master Mentes untied my wrists and ordered me to turn around and put my wrists behind my back. He tied my hands behind my back. He then reached over my shoulders and tied my boobs fairly tightly together at their base. My tits were even firmer than usual now. Their nipples quickly hardened. He pinched both nipples hard waking me from my dreamy state and making me yell. "What is my favorite color for your tits slave?" "Red sir." "You're darn right, especially if you're being punished. What do your tits exist for?" "To be played with and beaten sir." "Good girl."

Master Mentes then took out a short tit whip and proceeded to lightly whip my tits with it as I continued to kneel close to him but with my back to him. I closed my eyes instinctively but the whip never came anywhere close to my face. Master Mentes really knew how to whip tits. I could tell this was something he really enjoyed doing. He started playing with one of my nipples as he was whipping the other one. This whipping went on for about 15 minutes. He then put the whip down and took up the same slapper he had earlier used on my butt. He pulled my head back towards him by the hair exposing my breasts more and proceeded to spank them for real. *Slap, slap, slap, slap, slap, SMACK, SMACK, BAM, slap, slap.* Master Mentes concentrated spanking the fleshing mounds of the left breast, reaching out, grabbing it by the nipple, pulling it up and separating it from the right breast so more off my large breast was free to spank. It did sting but also felt sinfully good. "A forgetful, lazy slave girl needs to be a well beaten slave girl. Isn't that right slave*?"* *"Yess sir."* I managed to say. Smack...slap, slap, slap, SMACK, SMACK, BAM, slap. He pinched my left nipple as he held it making me wince but then he twisted it in-between his fingers giving me pleasure. He probably didn't even realize he was playing with the nipple in such a pleasurable way. Giving breasts pleasure and pain is just his nature. I sure wasn't going to complain. Then he let go of my left nipple and got a hold of the right nipple, pulling the right breast out to the right, separating it from its twin, allowing more of it to be beaten. Slap, slap, slap, SMACK, SMACK, BAM, slap. "Do you know how much I enjoy beating your tits slave?" *"Ow, oh...a lot sir."* "Girl do I ever." Slap, slap, slap, SMACK, SMACK, BAM, slap, slap. Blow after blow continued to rain down on my breasts, making them pink and tender. He pulled up my right breast by the nipple and concentrated his beating on the underside. It did hurt but frankly I got more pleasure from a tit whipping from him than when he spanks my ass. I glanced down at my breasts and they were getting red. He them grabbed both of my large nipples together with one hand and pulled my breasts up exposing their soft underbelly, going to work on them both at once with the slapper and spanking them hard now. *"Ow, ohh no sir, ow, oww, oh pleeaaseee."* Slap...slap, slap...slap, slap, SMACK, BAM...slap, slap. He let go of my tits and they flopped down. He then proceeded to spank their upper front. "You know how much I love spanking your tits" "yes sir, ow, ow, oh, ow." This was really hurting now and I wasn't going to be allowed to cum so I was going to just have to take it.

My breasts were now red and Master Mentes stopped. I thought my tit whipping was over but I was wrong. "Turn around slave." I turned around obediently and knelt there as he untied my wrists. Then in my stupor I remembered that there was another position for me and my tits to be whipped in...and more.

Master Mentes led me over to the half table. I was ordered to lay on my back on it. It was a familiar position for me. My pussy and ass were on the table's edge and thus would be easy to play with and take. My back and head were lying on the table. The ankles and thighs got tied to the stirrups. A strap came over my lower pelvis to keep it in place and straps held each arm in place. I was now quite vulnerable and immobile.

My master put me here often and left me here for his and other's pleasure. My legs are positioned such that my butt can be easily spanked and I could be taken in my ass. But for the time being Master Mentes was a lot more interested in finishing the job he started with my tits. Now though he would use the big black whip to beat them. This part would make me cry but leave my pussy dripping.

Master Mentes bent down to my pussy and sucked all the cum out of it. "You know what's coming now slave don't you." "Yes sir" I think I said. He raised the whip and CRACK. "Ow". CRACK, CRACK..SMACK. This is a big enough room so he could raise up the big whip and let it fly. *CRACK, CRACK...SMACK, BAM...SMACK, BAM.* I was now whimpering and trying to move away but to no avail. I was held too tightly in place and could go nowhere. BAM, SMACK, BAM. He was working up a sweat and loving every second of it. "Are you still going to be a forgetful slave?" "No sir". I was so exposed and I knew by now my pussy was dripping wet. I couldn't wait for him to take me in my ass like he always did. And he would take me for a long time too. I held onto that thought as the blows rained down on my chest. *"Please sir, oww, oww, ahhh."* Master Mentes was very skilled and the whip never landed more than a couple of inches above my breasts. Finally it was over but I kept crying.

He now played with my sensitive breasts grabbing, kneading, twisting, turning and holding them. "I am so proud of my work. Your breasts are so much fun to work with. You know your tits are my favorite tits to whip." Oh lucky me. "Thank you sir." I whimpered. He bent down and lightly bite my nipples one by one, also sucking on them and playing with my breasts more. He was so proud of his work and really did love my tits. Suddenly I remembered what was to come next, yes this would be great.

I looked down at my chest and it was a light shade of red. My nipples were hot and sensitive. I heard Master Mentes doing something and I looked over at him. His cock was hard and he was coming over to my exposed holes. First he got out some oil and used it and his finger to lubricate my anus. He inserted his finger deep into my ass making me moan in anticipation. He then cleaned off his finger. "Beg for it slave" he ordered. *"Sir please take me with your big, hard cock"*. "You can do better than that." *"Please sir I'm begging, please take me with your big hard cock and fuck me hard because I've been such a bad slave. I need to be fucked hard to clear my head and not be forgetful."* Satisfied he then entered my ass. Immediately I began begging to cum, which he allowed me to do.

Master Mentes grabbed my upper legs to hold me in place while he pounded my ass with his cock. I came so hard. I lost track of what time it was. "Come harder slut" he roared and I did just that pumping my hips against him as he took me. "You like how this feels in that naughty little ass of yours don't you slave." "Yes sir" I stammered. He pounded me harder and buried his cock all the way into my ass, just leaving it there for a few moments as he gyrated his hips, making it move from side to side. *"Ohhhhh sir, yes, thank you....ohhh."*

Master Mentes finished taking me a while later. He left me there tied down, exhausted and helpless. My tits were a light shade of red and my ass sore and tender. "I hope you will learn your lesson today slave but then again I hope you don't as I do love these sessions so much. Your owner said to leave you like this as Master Ponteus will be here soon to do as he wishes with you. What have you to say?" *"Thank you sir for disciplining and taking me."* "Good girl." With that he left.

Chapter Four

There I was alone and tied down waiting for the next person to punish and ravage me. It wasn't that big of a deal as I've been on this table like this often. I sure hope I don't have to go to the bathroom while no one is here though. Fortunately it's usually not a problem. Strapped down like this I could only move myself a bit from the tits up as my arms were strapped down which limited my movement.

Master Ponteus really liked to take me in the ass. A drawback to men in regard to the position I was strapped down to this table in, is that it is difficult for me to suck on their cocks. Mistresses can get on the table and sit on my face for me to pleasure them. Master Ponteus has had me in this position before so I was expecting the usual ass whipping and ass fucking. I didn't really like Master Ted that much and I don't think he's a particularly good lover but I had no say in the matter.

Then I heard someone enter, man I hope that's Master Ponteus, and I could tell from his voice that it was. "Wow, look at you. All ready to be beaten and taken." I wasn't sure if I was supposed to answer so I didn't say anything. I heard him undressing. "I'm going to fuck you silly slave. I heard about your forgetfulness and laziness, well I'm here to beat it right out of you." I heard noises like he was getting something together to spank me with. "Any requests for what I should spank you with?" "Your hand sir?" "Nice try but you know how I like my paddle." No not that paddle. He had a paddle that he had had for ages. The rustling I heard must have been him taking it off his cloths. He looked over and felt my ass. "How many spankings have you gotten today slave?" "Four so far sir." "Wow, your ass looks surprisingly good for all that, you always could take quite a spanking." "Thank you sir." He then came over and began playing with my tits, each hand on a tit. "Man I love these tits, especially when they are red like now. What do you say slave?" "Thank you sir." Getting my tits played with again felt good. They were still tender from the tit whipping though but gratefully were gifting me with pleasure. I started to groan seductively and move my head slowly back and forth. I knew he wouldn't let me cum so I didn't even try asking.

I heard some rustling then I felt him lubing up my anus for after the beating. Then suddenly I felt nothing. That's trouble. Past my upturn legs and exposed pussy I heard him beating the air with his paddle. Oh man, this is not good. Then he lightly swung the paddle against my ass many times. It was just the start of things to come. It would be my worst beating of the day so far. *SMACK, BAM, BAM...SMACK, SMACK, SMACK, BAM.* I yelled out from the beginning, making his cock hard no doubt. He grabbed my legs and drew himself closer to me. The beating continued. SMACK, SMACK, SMACK, BAM, BAM, BAM, BAM. I tried to move my ass but it was too securely in place. Then I realized I was crying *"Ow, ow, no please, ow, aw, aw, stop please, ohhh, nnnno."* He pulled my ass out as far as the pelvic strap would allow all in an effort to expose as much ass as possible. SMACK, SMACK, SMACK, BAM, BAM. Master Ponteus was in heaven, he is a sadistic man with permission to punish hard a wayward slave girl. I could not escape the blows that were raining down on my ass. *"I'mmm begging masterr, pleaseee."* BAM, SLAP, Slap, BAM...SMACK. Tears were running down my cheeks. I can usually take a good beating but as sensitive as my ass was from the days' previous onslaught and this brute of a master wailing away on my tender ass was too much. I don't think my owner would even be happy about this. I know this would leave plenty of marks on my ass. *"Masterrrr, pleaaaasse, oh, aw, pleassse stoppp pleaaaase, oh."*

Something on my ass felt different then I realized that the beating had stopped. Master Ponteus had also paddled my upper legs, something my owner will not like. Leaving marks on my legs, or on anyone else's property, is not good etiquette. I continued to cry. I didn't hear back from him but I heard him making himself harder and I knew the beating was over. He would concentrate now on my relaxed asshole. I felt him come up to me, grab both my hips and thrust himself into me..... *"ohhhh"* I shuttered glad to be feeling another type of sensation but my ass was still on fire.

Master Ponteus always grunted a lot when he fucked. It sounded real animal-like but a cock in my ass was a welcome change and soon I felt an orgasm coming on. Oh god, I hope this meany will let me cum. *"Permission to cum sir please."* No answer. *"Please sir may I cum….oh please, please."* I hate him. I tried hard to not cum and I was able to stifle the orgasm.

I don't get taken by him often and was going to talk to master about him, still his cock pounding my ass did feel good, even if I couldn't cum. I laid back and enjoyed it. At least 5 of my beatings for the day were over-with.

Chapter Five

I lay there on my back with my legs in the stirrups, exhausted. I remained strapped down to the table. I began reminiscing about the 5 hard spankings I'd had so far today. I knew I had 5 more to go, and as my ass and tits were quite tender and sore, I suspected those would be tough. I didn't know who else Master had invited to come punish me at this point but his good friend Master Adrēstos was certainly one.

I had been strapped down to this table for two long hard spankings, one of which included a tit whipping. Unfortunately nobody counts the tit whipping as a separate spanking which wasn't fair in my opinion. Master Ponteus, the last person to punish and take me while strapped down, had left me here, as did Master Mentes before him. I didn't mind being strapped down to the table terribly because it was comfortable and I had become tired from all the day's attention. So I dozed off to get some well deserved rest.

I was awakened a while later as much to my surprise, my very own wonderful owner walked in. He explained that he was taking the rest of the day off. He told me that he had been keeping up on my day's activity, then came over, inspected me and ran his hands over my lightly reddened breasts. "Wow, I bet your tits and ass are nice and tender by now." He inspected me further. "Well as you're so conveniently strapped down, I will now give you spanking #6."

Master went into his room and took off his clothes. Even though master is so strict and controlling, I must admit that I do love him and love serving him. He really does have my best interests in mind. I also love to see my master naked and it almost instantly turns me on. Master's ooze is so tasty and I frankly can't suck on his cock enough. If anything, master doesn't let me suck on his cock as much as I'd like. Hopefully I would have another opportunity real soon.

I didn't know what he had in mind for me. A lot depended on how horny he was. I already had a tit whipping, which was evident by my pink chest, so I didn't think he would give me that, at least until tonight. My guess was that with my strapped legs still in the air and my ass so easily accessible on the edge of the table, I would have at least the first part of spanking #6 here.

Master came over. "Eyes closed slave." I quickly shut my eyes but was saddened to have to lose sight of master.

The bad news is that he picked up a paddle and was heading my ass' way. "What have we learned about being forgetful in my house slave? Master said to me sternly. "That you won't tolerate it master." "Exactly."

Master was standing beside my ass now and massaging it roughly, he then pinched my redden globes many times. "Ow" I instinctively said. Master put a finger in my pussy to make sure I was wet. With the attention I just had, even though it was painful, I was still required to get wet. I did not let him down. Then much to my surprise master bent down and sucked on my wet pussy, I immediately begged to cum. *"Master pleassse may I...ohh may I cum?"* No answer, but there was no way I could stop from cumming if master is going to keep eating me for any length of time. *"Oh God please Master pleassse may I cummm?"* Thankfully he stopped. I exhaled then remembered master was still angry with me and standing next to my butt with a paddle. I guess you know what happened next. SMACK, SMACK, SMACK, SMACK, SMACK. *"Oh, ow, ohhhh, oh, master, oww."* Master really laid it on my butt, swinging hard and fast, SMACK, BAM, SMACK, SMACK, BAM, SLAP, SLAP, BAM. I was so strapped down that I couldn't move and had to just lay there with my already well spanked butt sticking out to take master' punishment. SMACK, SMACK, SLAP, SLAP, SMACK, BAM. Thank goodness master wasn't making me count the licks because he was spanking too fast and it really hurt now. I pulled on my arm restraints but it was no use. *"Owww, I'lll be ggood, owwwwwww, please master."* "What are you not going to do slave" master bellowed, breathing hard from spanking with so much vigor. "Be forgetful sir." Suddenly the spanking stopped. I had started crying and didn't even realize it. I probably got 80 stokes but since they were so fast I actually wasn't being spanked for that long. I don't think they were his hardest strokes either. Whatever the case was, once again my ass was on fire and I could do nothing about it. Master again bent down and sucked on my pussy, getting all the new pussy juice I created from the spanking.

Man that felt good. It almost made me stop feeling my raw butt, not quite though. All the spankings I would get now really would hurt with my ass being so tender.

I heard master doing something. I was concentrating so much on my scalding ass that I didn't see master getting ready to take me. But then I saw it and suddenly my butt didn't feel as bad. Usually master would take me for 20-30 minutes and man was I ever ready for it. Master entered my ass and immediately ordered me to cum. It guided effortlessly in. He then started to fuck his slave to his heart's content. He started slowly then started to really pound me.

Master' breathing got heavier and his grunting got more intense. *"Cum harder slave"* he ordered and I happily obeyed. I loved it when I helped make my master feel good like that and the events of the day I think are really turning him on. Master and his slave would soon feel quite sexually satisfied. Unfortunately for me, I knew that wasn't the last time master was going to beat me today. I did after all have 4 more spankings to go.

Chapter Six

Master took me for around 30 glorious minutes. Master finished exhausted. He re-gained his composure and unstrapped me from the table. Good thing because I had to go to the bathroom. I tried sitting but my butt wasn't ready for that so sat on a rolled up sheet of flax that I have used before for such occasions. Fortunately that helped. Man it's a good thing that I had such a tough butt. I went and laid down on my stomach but now I felt my tender tits. I turned over and lay on my back. That worked okay as long as I kept my legs up and most of the weight on my back.

Meanwhile Master had gone outside and was working. Maybe he'd forget I was there because usually in these situations, he'd put me in the cage.

Master had a cage custom built for me by a few of his warriors. It was in the playroom. The playroom had a dungeon like appearance. The walls had a number of hooks and racks preset into it as it was originally made. There was a number of different types of wooden horses for us slaves to be bent over and tied down to. I guess you can imagine what happens after that.

The cage could hold more than one slave at a time. It had a comfortable floor and a convenient opening on one side big enough for me to bend over and stick my ass through to the outside so folks can do whatever they wanted with it. With my ass sticking out of the cage in the manner I just mentioned, master would reach his hand into the cage and put a strap around my front pubic area to securely hold my butt out of the cage and in place. He would then beat my ass to his heart's content. Of course I could also be taken in that position. Often he would release me from that position, but keep me in the cage so he could come back later and do it again. I remember one time last moon I was whipped and taken off and on for half a day like that. It really hurt. Master Mentes had come by to also play with me. I would have been in the cage longer but master needed me to make dinner for them. While making dinner I would periodically have to lay over their laps for them to inspect me, play with me, spank me and run their hands and nails over my butt and tits. Master loved running his nails over my well spanked ass.

Master ordered me into his room. I knelt there for about 10 minutes. He then said it was time for my seventh spanking and this one he would give me while I was bent over and strapped to the wooden spanking horse in the playroom. He ordered me to go down and prepare it for my punishment. I said "yes master" and left, naked as the day I was born.

The wooden spanking horse was a great piece of equipment to spank a slave on. The slave's legs are spread to the sides of the horse and securely strapped to each side. The slave's ass is the highest point of her and her pussy and anus are readily available for use. An adaptation that master had made was that instead of the upper torso laying at the same angle *over* the other side of the horse, (thus the head bent over the horse and nearing the ground,) the upper body rested on a padded wood support that was parallel to the ground. At roughly the middle of the back was a strap to hold the upper body in place. Wrist straps held both arms in place at the wrist. There was a relatively wide hole for the slave's breasts to hang down through, thus making them readily available to play with or spank. With this set-up, the slave's tits and mouth were readily available for use. Another advantage to this adapted wooden horse set up from the slave's standpoint was that her butt cheeks weren't pulled so tight from the body being almost completely bent over. Maybe tighter butt cheeks hurt more, I didn't know for sure but thought so.

I could strap my legs down myself to save time, but master would have to strap my upper torso down, as well as both of my wrists. I will largely be immobile and completely vulnerable, just how I like it!

I heard Master approaching. I quickly turned my eyes away and looked down at the floor. "Good girl, you're ready to be fully strapped in." Master then strapped my torso down tightly with one strap and then strapped both my wrists down with the other two straps.

Master then went to the pile of implements and took out a big whip. The whips are my favorite thing to be beaten with. Maybe master didn't know that, though I had told him before. Maybe master was feeling a little bad about the extreme punishment I was enduring. Of course my ass was really sore already so this whipping would hurt plenty. Then...FLOP, and the whipping of slave Hera's ass started. *FLOP, CRACK, FLOP, BAM, CRACK, BAM, FLOP*. Master really got into it. I made some grunts but the truth was that the kind of pain this whipping *was* giving me, (and it was painful,) was okay. Still I'd better be careful and not need to cum or master will know it's not having the desired effect on me. Fine, I'll make like I'm hurting, then "OWWW!!!"

That's the problem with being whipped with your legs wide open like that, the pussy can take a direct hit, and just did. "Aw, did your pussy get hit. Here, I'll kiss it and make it feel all better." Master then bent down and sucked on my pussy. Wow, that made it feel better okay and immediately I needed to cum. "Please master may I cum?" "No." Master kept sucking on my pussy for about 30 seconds more, making me quiver. Then he reached down with his hand to tap on it instead, like he was thinking about spanking it. Gee I sure hope not, my pussy had escaped the spankings so far. It had been taken quite a bit today and frankly was a bit sore already. But master instead continued the whipping. *CRACK, FLOP, BAM, CRACK, BAM, FLOP*. I pulled on my wrist straps, like that was going to do me any good. *CRACK, BAM, FLOP*. The blows came down loudly and with a regular tempo, not hurting a lot but definitely getting my attention. I suspect master was starting to work up a sweat, something he would rather not do as he already bathed once today. Master then put down the whip and rubbed my butt. He bent down to suck up any more pussy juice I had made for him. He then went back to the pile to get another implement. "Oh yes, the small paddle. I haven't used that on your ass in at least a week." I looked over at him as he walked back to me swooshing the paddle in the air. He positioned himself off to the right of my ass...then...*CRACK, CRACK, CRACK*. "I haven't forgotten why you're here slave and will make sure your laziness is beaten out of you." "*Oww, ohh*" The paddle was landing on my upturned right cheek now in rapid succession, really hard too. I clenched my cheeks but that did no good. "I know that a well beaten slave is an attentive slave and you WILL be an attentive slave." At least 25 quick swats landed on my cheeks before he went to my left side and started the paddling again, this time concentrating on my left cheek. CRACK, CRACK, CRACK, BAM, BAM, SMACK, SMACK. I knew how wet my pussy had gotten and I could have cum if ordered to but I knew master was in no mood to let me cum. BAM, SMACK, CRACK, BAM, CRACK. The blows were now landing randomly all over my ass. Master started concentrating his blows on my upper legs. My thighs reddened faster than my ass for some reason and master liked that. Master then stopped long enough to suck up any new pussy juice I had made for him, the whipping then continued. "Count out the last 20 slave" he ordered. CRACK, *"onee"*, SMACK *"two master"*, BAM *"oh..three master"*, CRACK, *"oh, pleaseee, four master."* I counted out all 20 of the licks as ordered and just like that my spanking was done. Master rubbed my hot, sore ass. "We both know how tough it is to get marks to stick on your ass and I am so happy to see your ass so marked up. For days you slave will be reminded every time you sit down of the importance of not being forgetful." "Yes master." I managed to say. My ass really hurt and I had been crying but I was sure to shed copious amount of tears before this day was over. He kept rubbing my ass. "And to think there are 3 more spankings to go" he said happily.

Soon I stopped crying but softly moaned, wiggling from the pain as I continued to lay strapped down to the horse wishing so much that I could rub myself.

Chapter Seven

I continued to lay over the horse helpless and vulnerable, waiting to be further used and abused. I looked over at Master who was sitting against a wall. I waited for a moment, then when I thought he wasn't concentrating on something, I spoke. "Master" I meekly blurted out. "Yes slave" he said. "Would 10 spankings in one day be the most you ever have given to a slave in your life?" He didn't need to think and quickly answered "Yes." "Well it sure will be a personal best for me." We both had an uncomfortable laugh. There was a pause. "I've had too many problems over the years from your laziness and you know that. This is just the first day should that continue to be a problem." I swallowed hard. Oh man that didn't sound good. I mean I've cum a lot today but my ass was really hurting and I had 3 spankings left.

Master then got up, came over and turned the horse I was strapped to so my ass, pussy and anus were directly facing him while he sat. I must have made a great sight. He could also see my breasts dangling towards the ground.

I wiggled a bit to adjust myself in the straps. About 15 minutes later, abruptly master came over, bent down and sucked on my pussy. Wow. With each hand he grabbed an asscheek and squeezed hard. I let out a yell. "Cum for me slave" he yelled and man did I ever. "Ohhhhhh." With each hand he started lightly spanking each cheek, sucking like crazy. This day really must have turned master on as I don't get eaten by his a real lot but he was looking for as much pussy juice as possible and clearly did not think I was giving him enough. "Is that all the pussy juice you're going to give me? Fine, I think we can change that." Man that didn't sound good. He went and got a black leather slapper and started once again sucking but this time while pounding my ass with the slapper. *"Oh owww. I'lll cummm haaarder."* Master then dug his fingernails into my bruised ass cheeks. That made me scream. *"AWWWW".* He sucked so hard that it hurt but I came as hard as I could and know I gave him a mouthful because the spanking stopped and the eating continued. Several minutes later master stopped, contented.

"Master" I asked, "does that count as one spanking?" "No such luck Hera." Well it was worth a try. All the spankings now were really going to hurt and I knew it. Then I heard Master Adrēstos at the front doorway. Master looked at me and said *"Good news spanking number 8 is minutes away."* Good news for who? I squirmed and felt a shiver go down my spine.

Master Adrēstos was a stout man who like Master Mentes, loved my breasts. He's played with me before while I was in this position. No doubt he would sit in front of me and play with my tits for a while. Like Master Mentes he loved my breasts. Everybody loved my breasts. I felt a bit of a chill on my sore ass. I hoped I wouldn't cry from my next spankings but I figured I would. My last one or two spankings of the day would be by master and I figured he would let me have it good. He just loves giving me a good spanking.

I heard the two of them come over and Master Adrēstos immediately commented on my marked red ass. "Wow, this ass looks great. Man, I can't wait to add to that." I shook for a moment with anticipation. Master Adrēstos took off his cloths. Now everybody in the room was naked, only I was the only one tied down and helpless. He came over to me while making small talk with my owner and started caressing my beaten ass and upper thighs. It felt good. "I hope you've been learning your lesson." "Yes sir. I have learned my lesson." Both masters had a short laugh from that remark.

As I predicted, Master Adrēstos sat down in front of me and started playing with my breasts. My breasts, though still sore, were not near as sore as my ass. His hands really felt good though. He then took out a container of olive oil, put a big glob on each hand and commenced to massage my breasts using the lubrication of the oil. That always felt good. My owner would do that too. Within 60 seconds I was ready to cum. I asked for permission and got it. My master then went back to my pussy and started eating me again. Oh my God did I ever cum. I know I gave him lots of pussy juice. With his fingers, Master Adrēstos ran circles around the lubricated fleshy part of my breasts for many minutes making me beg to have my nipples played with. *"Master Adrēstos please play with my nipples so I can give my owner more pussy juice."* That was the way to ask as he suddenly did and my body shook from the intensity of the orgasm. "Awwwwwww yessssss, awwwwww." Waves of pleasure rolled over me and I strained at my bonds as the spasms engulfed me. *"Awwwwww."* 10 minutes of this came and went, still master was eating me, then he stopped eating me and went back to his seat. The breast massage would also end a few minutes later. What a divine interlude it was.

Master Adrēstos cleaned off the oil from my breasts and his hands. He then got closer to me and pushed his cock into my mouth. I sucked for all I was worth. The longer I sucked after all, the longer before my next my spanking would start. After 10 or so minutes of that, which made my mouth somewhat tired actually, he went to his bag and pulled out a wooden paddle. Looks like the business of the day was at hand.

"So your forgetfulness has returned slave?" "Yes sir" I reluctantly admitted. "Definitely that needs to be addressed immediately." With that he went behind me and rubbed the paddle over my butt, then WHACK. I jumped, oh that hurt. WHACK, WHACK, WHACK. "Ow, owww, pleaseee noo." WHACK, WHACK, WHACK. I strained at my bonds and my torso jumped up sending my breasts bouncing up. SMACK, BAM, WHACK, WHACK. *"Nooo..I..won't forgettt."* BAM, WHACK, WHACK, slap, slap. The paddling went on for what seemed very long and I finally broke down and cried, much to the delight of everybody. *"Oh, please sir, no pleassee."* Tears were now running down my cheeks as the pain was intense. Master Adrēstos was spanking my thighs now, including the middle thighs that had earlier been left unscathed. Back to my ass he went pounding away without mercy. *"Oh god, nooo please..."* I begged. Then my owner intervened. He wanted more of his slave's pussy juice. All I knew was that the spanking had stopped and master was coming over. Once again he bent down and sucked on my pussy looking for more pussy juice from his slave. My ass hurt so much now though that I couldn't cum and was grateful that nobody ordered me to. My owner had his fill and now sat down in front of me pushing his cock into my mouth. I immediately sucked away on it for all I was worth. In the meantime, Master Adrēstos had exchanged the paddle for a strap and my beating once again continued, though not as hard out of respect for my master who had his cock in my mouth. SMACK, SMACK, BAM, WHACK, WHACK. *"Owww"* I began letting out a continuous muffled scream. The blows came down very fast. Master Adrēstos was not messing around but still I had to force myself to pleasure my master or the beating would never end. I sucked on my owner's cock as hard as I could, forcing my mind to concentrate on just that, not my scalding ass. *WHACK, WHACK, BAM, BAM, CRACK, CRACK.* Both masters were clearly getting so much pleasure from my ordeal that I could not tell when it would stop. Just then Master Adrēstos stopped and went and got another paddle, a big one with holes in it. "And for the finale, ten of my best." My master took his cock out of my mouth and sat back contentedly watching. "Count them out slave." BAM" *"Ahhhh, one sir."* BAM " *Oww two sir."* SMACK *"owww three sir."* I was crying hard now and even when the paddle wasn't landing on my ass it still hurt. It all felt like one continuous intense spanking. I kept counting out the blows though and finally they ended but my crying continued on. I pulled on my bonds, and as usual that did no good. I would continue crying for ten minutes after the spanking ended. Both masters sat down and chatted, very impressed with themselves. In time I heard Master Adrēstos get up. I looked back and watched him lube up my anus. He then made himself hard and entered me in it.

Master Adrēstos grabbed me by the sides and pounded me from the beginning. I was still sniveling but soon, gratefully, a wave of pleasure rolled over me and I begged for permission to cum. My master allowed it. Wow did I ever need that. With my ass so sore, sorer than it's ever been, I needed to get my mind on something else. My owner came over and once again stuck his cock in my mouth. I sucked as hard as I could. Master then unstrapped my wrists so I could play with his balls. I concentrated on my master' cock, sucking as hard as I could. I was now cumming hard and not concerned about my scalding ass.

I don't know how long all that lasted but in time there was no cock in my ass and my owner went back to my pussy for a reload of my pussy juice. I hope I once again was giving him all he wanted but I don't really know. I was left there exhausted and limp as the both masters got dressed and chatted. I heard something about me but couldn't make it out. My master came over and unstrapped me and ordered me into the big cage were I obediently went, rubbing my ass furiously. I looked back at my ass after I was locked securely in the cage and saw it was dark red with more marks. Tell me I didn't really have 2 more spankings to go. This was definitely the day from Hades. Both masters went outside and left me naked with my thoughts and well-beaten tits and ass.

Chapter Eight

The best I could do was lie down on my side in the cage. Sitting was no longer an option. I hoped that one of my next beatings would be on my tits as they were in less pain than my ass. Soon master came down, opened the cage and ordered me to make dinner. I had stopped crying and was ready for a change. I was ordered to stop as I walked by so he could rub my scorching ass. "Wow" he exclaimed. "I don't think I've ever seen it like this." "It hurts terribly master. Please no more. I have learned my lesson I swear." I did really feel I had learned my lesson. It didn't however phase him.

My master was in the main room drinking a glass of wine. Master Adrēstos had left a while back. I was cooking dinner in the fireplace in the main room. I asked my owner "Master do I really need any more spankings today?" He smiled and said "yes you do slave, but I will be giving both of them to you." I think that was good. At least I knew his style better. He then added "The last spanking of the night will be your bedtime spanking but the second to the last you can choose. It can be spanking your tits, or your ass. You think about which you'd prefer." "Yes master." Well the answer was easy, spank my tits. They didn't hurt as much and hopefully I could get some pleasure from it. I blurted out "spank my tits please sir." "Very well."

I fixed dinner and ate with master. During dinner, amazingly my spankings never came up. We made small talk. I cleared the table, cleaned the dishes outside and went back to the main room and into master' arms. I was naked of course as master was.

It was about 7:30 and master kissed me and said it was time for my tits to get the required attention. I said yes master and dragged myself up. We both went to the playroom. "You pick what I shall use on them and come here with it." "Yes sir" I said obediently. I went to the pile of implements and looked around. Well gee, from experience I knew the pig leather slapper hurt my ass the least so let's try that. I brought it to master who was sitting against a wall smiling. He had rope with him and ordered me to sit in front of him with my hands behind my back. I forced myself to sit on my butt, he then tied my wrists together so they'd be behind my back and out of the way.

To my surprise master then ordered me to sit in front of him, thus I would be on the same level as him. He took out oil and before I knew it my breasts were getting massaged like Master Adrēstos had earlier. At first they were sensitive from the whippings of the day but the pain subsided and turned into some type of painful pleasure. I cooed and rubbed my back seductively up against my master's chest as waves of pleasure emanated from my breasts. They were always so sensitive and my owner loved them. It took me longer than usual but I finally asked for permission to cum. I came quietly. Master would concentrate on the nipples for a while, running his lubricated fingers quickly in circles around them, then pull back to knead and massage all of both breasts, while trying not to touch the nipples. Then all of a sudden he would furiously twist around the more sensitive and now very slippery nipples, which would make me explode with pleasure. Master went on and on with this and I kept cumming for him, admittedly not my hardest orgasm of the day but a very welcome sensation. Then master pulled me out of my haze by stopping. He cleaned his hands and my tits off with a cloth that he had handy, then he ordered me to sit with my back to him on the ground just below him. Sitting was still a tough experience but I had the pillow of rolled up flax under me which helped. Master pulled my head back towards his lap and ordered me to keep it there so as to have a better spanking angle on my breasts. He took up the slapper and ran it over my breasts for some time, massaging them with it. I quivered in anticipation. Then the spanks started but only light ones and they stayed light for some time, though progressively getting stronger. Master concentrated spanking both nipples, but clearly this was meant not to be a hard spanking. I had gotten lucky. Master would grab a nipple and pull the breast up and out, that way it gave him more tit to spank. He did this with both breasts several times. With the breast pulled out by the nipple, he would concentrate spanking its lower breast, then both sides of that breast and then the upper breast. Clearly master was really enjoying himself. My tits were already rather red and this made them redder. It did hurt though as they were already beaten hard twice today. After 60 or so light to moderate spanks to my tits, it was over. Master untied me, turned me around and pulled me over for a kiss. He sat me next to him for more cuddling and talk. He did warn me though that my last spanking of the day, my bedtime spanking, would be a hard one and that I would cry myself to sleep tonight.

Chapter Nine

As master and I shared some quiet time together, he had me suck on his cock for around 15 minutes. He was particularly horny that day as I've noted. He later had me get down on the carpet in front of him. He then tied my wrists together behind me then had me kneel in front of him so he could more readily play with my breasts. He would reach down from time to time to massage and lightly spank my upturned bottom with a long stick. He wasn't spanking hard at the moment but I knew that would come later, and sure enough it did. In the meantime though master provided me with a good helping of his delicious ooze. He then told me that the finale of the day was at hand. He untied my wrists, I was then ordered to get ready for bed. My instructions were to lay face down on my belly waiting for my 10th and final spanking of the day. I had butterflies in my stomach because I knew how hard this spanking would be. Still I was grateful that I had had so much pleasure that day and also had provided others, particularly my wonderful master, so much pleasure. Still I knew what was coming up would be really tough and I knew master wanted it to be that painful so I would cry myself to sleep. Knowing that such a severe spanking was eminent in a way was good because I would know not to hold back and to instead start crying as early as I wanted too.

I did my nighttime routine and told master I was ready for bed. Master ordered me to kneel in front of him so he could tie my hands together in front of me. I was naked as usual, now with my hands tied in front of me. I got onto my bed on my stomach and waited for what was sure to be a very painful experience.

I was genuinely scared and quite unexpectedly I started to cry while just waiting for this terrible punishment. Master came in with a leather strap and a paddle. He sat down next to me and began sternly lecturing me. He was clearly working himself up to do something sadistic. I apologized profusely for being forgetful as I was crying already out of fear. Then he began spanking me.

I would cry the entire time. Master doesn't usually spank me with his hand but today was an unusual day in many respects. SMACK, SMACK, BAM, WHACK, WHACK. *"Owww"* I let myself go and cried with abandon, more than I really needed. I had really let my master down and I deserved this punishment, I knew that. His blows came down very fast. CRACK, CRACK, BAM, BAM, BAM, WHAP, WHAP. "I am absolutely not accepting your forgetfulness anymore and will happily have it beaten out of you." *"Owww, yesss sir, oh, pleassee noo more."* SMACK, BAM, WHACK, CRACK, CRACK, BAM. Master then went back and forth spanking each cheek as hard as he could for around 5 minutes. He was genuinely upset. He took up the strap and while holding me down, and without hesitation, once again began beating. *"Nooo ohh...masters....oww...ahhh...ahhh."* My ass was once again on fire and really hurting. I was hoping it would turn me on enough to cum but no way. WHAP, WHAP, WHAP, CRACK. He apparently grew tired for the moment of beating my ass and used the strap on my upper thighs, now grunting at times as he laid down the blows. I was no longer feeling the individual spanks as much and instead it all melded into one continuous wave of pain. I tried to turn my ass away from the blows but the combination of his strong grip and the tight bondage made that impossible. He continued to lay it on my ass with abandon. WHACK, WHACK, CRACK, WHAP. *"Ow, ohhh, owww, no, pleaseee..ahhhh."* I bent my head back and clenched my buttcheeks with all my might but it did no good. Master was hell bent on taking care of this problem once and for all.

This spanking no doubt hurt worse thanks to all the spankings I already had. I was laying on my sore tits but quickly I would not be feeling their soreness, even though I was rubbing them against the flax sheets as I wiggled back and forth. CRACK, WHAP, WHAP, SLAP, WHAP. My crying was uncontrollable now and bordered on a wail. This is what my master wanted. This was a big time spanking that we would talk about for years to come and that he would threaten me with if I was bad. *"Owww, no, ahhhh, stoppp pleassee."* It went on and on and master was breathing heavy now, still angrily scolding me off and on but I could no longer tell what he was saying. My mind was in a heavily spanked haze. I didn't dare look at my ass but I knew this would leave lots of marks and sitting would be difficult for many days. SMACK, SMACK, CRACK, WHAP, WHAP. I kicked my feet as much as I could. I kept clenching my cheeks but when I would do that master would beat the cheeks harder. Then he stopped but I knew it was just to get the paddle for the last round of this nightmare. I would never be forgetful, I just couldn't go through this again. I must work harder. Master grabbed me around the waist once again and without a word began where he left off. Now the blows from the paddle were aimed for the top of the left cheek, where it meets the back and steadily landing further and further down until 30 or so spanks later it was on the middle thigh. He then did the same to the right cheek. I had lost touch with space and time and was crying like I never had from a spanking. I don't remember what I said as I pleaded for him to stop, and then it was over.

Master threw down the paddle and got up and walked off. I lay there sobbing. *"I'llll never dooo it again."* I promised. I wanted so badly to rub my ass but couldn't as my hands were tied together too securely. Unfortunately for me the torment continued as my ass was in so much pain. 10 minutes later I tried to stop crying but couldn't. 30 minutes later master would come back and sit down beside me. I pleaded for his forgiveness. He rubbed my bottom lovingly. "I do this because I care so much for you Hera." I tried to thank him but was having too much trouble talking. I managed to mumble something. Master rubbed my cheeks. My hands however he left tied knowing that now I still couldn't rub my cheeks, which was something I wanted to do so badly. He pulled the covers over me, kissed my cheek and left the room, leaving me alone with my thoughts and incredibly sore ass. I kept on crying and sure enough cried myself to sleep.

The End

This book is sold and/or distributed with the understanding that the publisher and author is not engaged in rendering legal or other professional services. **This book and its subject matter are for entertainment purposes only.** In this publication there may be inadvertent inaccuracies including technical inaccuracies, typographical inaccuracies and other possible inaccuracies. **The writer and publisher of this publication expressly disclaim all liability for the use or interpretation by anybody of information contained in this publication.** The author, publisher and distributors of this publication hereby disclaim any and all liability for any loss or damage caused by errors or omissions resulted from negligence, accident, or any other causes. If legal advice or other expert assistance is required, the services of a competent professional person in a consultation capacity should be sought. Products, services and websites' content vary with time. Please verify any published information.

Book #7 - Fourteen Male-Female Anal Sex Stories

By Jennifer S.

Copyright (C) 2013

Fourteen Male-Female Anal Sex Stories

1. My name is Erica. I'm a 114 lb pretty Mexican lady with straight black hair and full lips. My breast size is 32C. I was particularly proud of my firm very well proportioned ass that was perfect for playing with, and other things.

It was the morning on the 16th of December and as is the norm on weekdays I got on a very crowded subway to go to work. I was wearing a short black dress. I had black stockings on as well as black bra and panties. It was winter so I also wore a coat.

I was lucky enough to catch the express train even though it was packed. Nearly 15 minutes into the 45 minute ride I felt something brush against my ass as I stood holding onto the rail in the middle of the subway car. Then it happened again. Touching my ass is a huge turn on for me and I was still sleepy so I not only didn't get concerned about it but actually got turned on by it. Still I had forgotten about it when it happened a 3rd time. It was so crowded but I still tried turning around. I got a glimpse of a great looking guy looking down on me and standing right behind me. I knew it was him. He had a tie on and looked like an executive. He had a friendly but firm face. Then he leaned against my butt and now I was feeling his cock inside his pants. Suddenly the subway car went into a turn that forced my ass further into the cock. Suddenly I felt nothing and for the next 5 minutes I was horny as hell just thinking about what had just happened. If there was room I wanted to turn around and see what happened to him but what if he was gone and there was someone else there? What if I thought it was him but it was somebody else. I was very nervous but really turned on. Nothing like this had ever happened to me before.

Suddenly, a man whispered in my ear to stay still, not make a sound, and enjoy it. Soon I felt a hand on my so spankable ass slowly working its way down and under my skirt targeting my panties. Fingers went inside my panties and down the crack of my ass to my asshole. The next thing I knew my asshole was being taken by a lubricated finger, a long one too. The finger rammed my anus and stopped me right in my tracks. I was so turned on I didn't want to turn around or say anything that could interfere with this adventure, besides I love to have my asshole played with as much as I love to get taken in it.

My ass was being finger fucked by a pro for seemingly an eternity. He was very deliberate. He started out slowly then took me very fast then rested with slow thrusts and went back to fast pumping. Oh my gosh, what if I came right there in the subway car. It was so crowded and loud that if I was quiet nobody was likely to even notice, but suddenly it stopped and his delicious finger had partially been taken out of my ass. I stood there hoping for more, then, before I could turn around, my invader suddenly drove his finger in as far as it could go and left it there for the remainder of the ride, wiggling it regularly.

It was the most exciting subway ride I've ever had. While his finger rested inside of me I decided to try and cum. I closed my eyes and inconspicuously fucked his finger and sure enough had a nice, quiet orgasm as I held tight to the overhead rail so I wouldn't fall incase my knees buckled.

Then as we approached a stop, I felt his finger pull out of me. I wanted to turn around in case he wanted to get to know me better but was too shy to.

I arrived at the office and was horny the entire day. Later that evening I put my two vibrators to very good and lengthy use.

Every day I got on the subway at the same time looking for him. It was frustrating in a sense, but I really wondered what he was like and fantasized about having a date with him. Was he a great lover? Would he only want to take me in my ass?

I had given up on finding what in my mind I had somehow made into my dream man, when a week later I got on the subway to work and there he was. The subway wasn't as crowded then and even though I relished the thought of him finger fucking my ass again, it would be tougher to hid, besides there was an open seat next to him so I sat there. Would this be my only chance to get to know him better?

I couldn't ask him if he was the guy that played with my asshole like that as what if he wasn't. He could also be afraid to admit to it as he may be afraid he could get in trouble. He wasn't starting the conversation so I worked up the courage and asked him for the time. He was friendly and gave it to me and thankfully the conversation developed. We even agreed to meet for drinks later that day but my ass being finger fucked hadn't yet come up.

Well anyway I now live with him and yes that was him. Now he enjoys my asshole in many other ways and whenever he wants.

2. My boyfriend is the type who likes to fuck me in my ass, but still prefers to fuck my pussy, so I don't get it in the ass a real lot. I on the other hand love it in the ass. Therefore, I got pretty excited when Kevin called and said he was coming over to take me in the ass and I shouldn't have anything on, be on the bed waiting for him and already be well lubed. How nice, tonight I would have a little delicious pain and A LOT of pleasure.

30 minutes or so later he arrived. He had a key to my apartment so he walked right into the bedroom where I was eagerly waiting for him. His cloths were off in a flash and he sat down in front of me on the bed where I eagerly sucked on his cock. After 5 minutes of sucking, he lifted my head off of him and told me on to get on my hands and knees. He dried his hard cock off with a small towel so the condom would stick, put the condom on, lubed it, then entered my very ready ass.

"Does it hurt?" Kevin asked me, sliding another couple inches into me. I replied by shoving my ass back against him and taking the rest of his pulsing cock into my tight hole. His moans of pleasure told me that he was enjoying it too. He cautiously began pumping his cock in and out. I could tell he was concerned about hurting me. But as I'm the impatient type, I started pushing myself back into him, getting him to fuck me harder and faster. "Ooh yes" he said. "I'm going to cum in your tight little ass!"

That comment sent me over the edge, and I orgasmed long and hard. Just as I was finishing, I felt splashes of hot cum shooting deep inside my ass. It felt amazing, and it made me cum again.

Well this now has become a regular part of our playtime.

3. It was my boyfriend's birthday, and as well as a gift of a great shirt, I decided to give him another more personal present, my ass.

My name is Cindy and I'm a 29 year old brunette. 125 lbs, 5'3", 38 B boobs. Brad and I had been dating for a couple of months. He wanted to take me in my ass but I resisted it as I'd never experienced such a thing before. He had put toys in my ass when playing with me, and often when he was taking me doggie style, he would put a dildo in my lubricated ass which was attached to his body via a cord which was wrapped around his waist. Thus when he thrust into me, his pelvis pushed both his cock into my pussy as well as the dildo into my ass. It was great to be on my hands and knees with both of my holes being filled!

A few days ahead of time I told him on the phone about the special birthday present I was giving him, and I must admit that the anticipation was killing me. I couldn't wait. If I liked it I'd want us to do it a lot more often.

The night arrived and after a small birthday gathering at a bar, we returned for the main event.

Our clothes were off in a flash. I told him how I just couldn't wait for him to take me in my ass and how I had been thinking about it all week. He thought this would be a very memorable birthday present.

With my pussy at the edge of the bed, he ate it like it was dessert. With his birthday present in mind I gifted him with lots of pussy juice. He then told me to get further up on the bed and get on my elbows and knees. The moment was not far off. He then lubed my anus up pushing the lubrication deep and spending a lot of time finger fucking me. Little did he know how ready I was for this anal treat. He then sat against the head board and had me lay down on my stomach in front of him and make his cock hard with my mouth. I sucked away on his cock, sucking down his ooze as I made his cock harder and harder. I loved to feel a cock hardening in my mouth and clearly he was really enjoying himself too. Then suddenly he lifted my head off of his cock. The moment of truth had arrived.

He got behind me and oh my god I got entered! He started pumping my ass in a slow and deliberate motion. Like I envisioned all week, I loosened my anus as much as I could, and that seemed to make all the difference in the world. I figured I'd enjoy finally being taken in the ass and I did! Though I guess it helps to be so turned on.

Well that was a while back and being taken in the ass is a regular occurrence now. When we're having sex, Tom starts in my pussy and finishes in my ass!

4. The long and short of it is that I screwed up and accepted that my husband had the right to punish me. I would have preferred the usual spanking but he's done that so much with me over the years that mainly it just turns me on, so he thought of another punishment. I would have to wear a butt plug all day. He would put it on before we went to work and after we both got home he would take it out, at a time of his choosing. (We work at the same place in the garment district in Los Angeles. We had good jobs thanks to it being his family's business.)

He had put butt plugs in me before at different times for significant periods, such as when I was doing housework. Only on one other occasion however did I leave the house with a butt plug in me. It was once when I drove to the supermarket, with a stopover at the gas station for a fill-up, (of gas that is.)

I would have protested but I didn't know what other nasty punishment he would then do to me instead. (He can be very mischievous when it comes to punishing me.)

A very important part of this punishment was going to be which butt plug I would have to "wear". We had several. We had one he called the "spreader". It was 5 inches long and 1½ inches at its thickest point. There was one that was 6 inches long and an inch at its thickest. It looked like a penis and vibrated (mmmmm.) There is also the butt plug he called "ole reliable." It was 4 1/2" long and tapers to 1" at its widest. Then there were the anal beads. (As you can tell my asshole gets a lot of attention when it comes to sex.) He chose one of the anal beads.

Tomorrow would be Wednesday and that was determined to be the fateful day. Tomorrow came along and he picked my clothes out for me. I would be wearing a dark brown skirt, one of my stronger pairs of white panties (with an extra one in my purse just in case,) a white bra and a white button down blouse.

With just my bra on I put on my make-up then bent over a chair and waited as my husband came over, lubed me up well and inserted the anal bead toy well into my ass. Then using lots of white cloth first aid tape, he taped my asshole securely shut. After a quick spanking, we continued getting ready and I got in the car with him (often we take separate cars) but not today as he was having too much fun watching me fidget in my seat.

I would be allowed to lubricate my anus as much as I wanted throughout the day but I never did. If I was sitting I could pivot into a comfortable position. The bending down to sit could really get my attention. Getting up and walking was a different story and as the day progressed it made for some interesting moments.

Twice my husband called me down to the warehouse where he worked, to watch me walk. When no one was watching he had me bend over with my butt in front of him. Bending over was something I had to be very careful doing as the dildo stuck out a bit that way even though my muscles, the tape and my underwear mostly kept it in place. He had fun pushing it in even though it would quickly pop back towards him a bit. It also got me so turned on.

Still my anus felt raw after we got home and my husband finally took it out. But the sex that night was mind blowing!

5. I was on my hands and knees and Tom was kneeling behind me.

I found myself saying "Oh yes! I want more of you in me. I want you to finger fuck me like I've never been fucked before." I felt Tom slide yet another finger inside my pussy, then, without warning his lubricated, well manicured thumb entered my tight ass. I cried out and began bucking my hips against his hand. It hurt a bit but oh it felt so good.

"Oh god, fuck me hard." I felt Tom rocking his hand back and forth and up and down. First his fingers thrust into my pussy then his hand pulled out and up so his thumb could thrust even further into my ass. He pumped his finger in my ass all the while fucking my pussy with his other fingers. "Oh god yes! That feels so good!"

"What am I doing to you baby? Tell me."

"You're fucking my pussy with your fingers, and fucking my ass with your thumb."

Just then, Tom pulled out a finger in my pussy and also stuck it in my ass along with his thumb. Then he furiously fucked both my holes. "Now you've got two fingers in my ass. Yes, fuck me harder! Faster!"

I felt myself tightening up and Tom must have felt it also as he fucked my pussy and ass hard after slowing a bit for a rest. I exploded onto his hand and began bucking my hips against him. The orgasm I had was so intense, I heard myself ask him to stop, but I didn't mean it. I moaned and screamed, and suddenly I came again. In time Tom pulled his hand out of both my holes.

All I could do was lay there, completely exhausted. "Did you enjoy that baby?" Tom asked softly.

"Mmmmmmmmmmmmmmmmmmmmmmmm" I replied as Tom kissed me tenderly before walking away.

6. My husband bought me a fucking machine for Christmas. It was an amazing surprise that I never expected. He goes on the road a significant amount so for that reason alone it would come in handy. Needless to say it got used often, which doesn't help our electricity bill!

One night though it was used on me for something unexpected, for punishment. I had forgotten to pay some bills which caused some problems to our credit rating. It was just a case of being forgetful and my husband wanted to nip that in the bud.

That night, at dinner, he informed me that my punishment tonight would be to be taken in the ass by the spanking machine, and only in the ass. We had tried anal sex before but I found it hurt but after screwing up our credit rating I found myself in no position to argue, and if anything felt I needed to be punished.

An hour or so after dinner, Jim told me to strip and wait for him next to the machine. I was nervous and even trembled from time to time. I knew Jim wanted to take me in my ass more often but it hurt, besides I exercised my pussy good and hard to make sure it was nice and tight for him.

Soon he came over and told me to "assume the position". I got on my elbows and knees at the usual spot and distance from the machine's arm that had the dildo at its end.

He didn't waste anytime either. He slowly slid the machine's dildo up into my ass. Even though it was thoroughly lubricated, it took a bit of time before it was finally stuffed all the way up my ass. I tried to ignore it and I hoped I would find it more comfortable later on. He then got up and went to the kitchen to get a drink.

When he came back I knew the time had come. There is a manual control lever on the fucking machine so one can manually make the machine's arm go back and forth; he activated that and my ass began to officially be taken.

He started slow and it made me moan. It did hurt some but starting slow like this was real helpful. I put my head down and loosen my asshole as much as I could.

What I really wanted to be able to do is cum from it. Also I knew that Jim at some point would sit in front of me and I'd be sucking on his cock while my ass was being taken.

"Keep your butt in place" he said. I didn't realize it but I was moving away some so less and less of the dildo was entering me. I quickly straighten out. Then Jim let the machine take over by turning it on.

The noise of the machine startled me but that ended up being a momentary concern. The fact is that fucking my ass was indirectly working my clit, even if my anus was the hole furthest from it.

The good news is that I was feeling okay and things would get better still as suddenly I heard the unmistakable humming of a vibrator next to me. Jim ran the vibrator along my pussy slowly then more quickly, and that would be the end of my fear of being taken anally!

"Oh yes, please, more…" Was that me that said that? Wow, it was. I actually was now humping the fucking machine and felt my first orgasm coming on. "Ohhhhhhhhh." I put my head down and just hollered, "Oh god yes…more…" I came all over that vibrator and know my ass being fucked had a lot to do with it.

Jim then took away the vibrator and told me I had to cum from the ass fucking alone. I wanted so much to do that and knew I could. He got in front of me and sure enough I was sucking on his cock while my ass was being taken by the machine. It was amazing. He reached down and played with my boobs too. I now had two of my holes filled and my boobs being played with, but still no orgasm. 10 or so minutes later I was not only rewarded for all my sucking efforts with a mouth full of my husband's cum but I also came along with him as well!

Well I now often get taken by the fucking machine like that night, sometimes in my pussy, sometimes in my ass and sometimes in my pussy and then ass. Assuming my husband's home during that time I usually have his cock in my mouth, sucking the daylights out of it.

What a punishment that turned out to be!

7. After my boyfriend Joe spends some time fucking my pussy, it's time to take me in my ass. As part of foreplay he has already lubed my tight hole. He slowly puts his cock into my very tight asshole. It feels so tight going in but once it's in there, it feels incredible. Sometimes Joe fucks my ass really fast and sometimes he starts slow. I'll be moaning the whole time. I play with my clit and/or use a vibrator on my wet pussy. I fuck my pussy with my hand while Joe fucks my ass. His thrusts are very deep and very hard. We both love it so. Joe will spank me while taking me in my ass. It stings some but feels so good.

8. After watching TV in bed my husband and I decide to fuck, so we take off the rest of our clothes. After I suck on his cock to make it hard, my husband told me to get on my hands and knees. He then guides his very hard, thick cock into my dripping wet cunt. He thrusts deeper and deeper and it feels so incredible.

Soon his hands are all over my boobs and I turn my head and lean back so we can kiss deeply and passionately. He grabs my ass and starts to spank it, first lightly but the swats keep getting harder and harder and that feels great too. No words are usually spoken while we are lost in our hot, wild sex.

At some point my husband reaches for the lube and applies it to my tight hole, who's turn to be taken has come. He slowly glides his cock into my ass. I gasp a little at first from the delicious pain but he takes his time. At first he enters me slowly, but soon really starts to fuck my tight ass. He spanks my cheeks which make them a little sore but it feels great to be spanked while I'm being fucked in the ass. The thrusts are so deep and while he is fucking my sweet ass I am fucking my pussy with my fingers. I'm so wet that my pussy cums all over my fingers. I then take my fingers out of my wet cunt and let my husband taste them. He licks all the cum up and continues to fuck my ass harder and faster. Eventually he cums in my ass with a shout.

9. I love to ride Craig while Jon fucks me in the ass. I didn't like ass play until recently but I gave into their persistent requests as they told me they would be gentle and make me love it by the time we're finished. I start by straddling Craig and ride him with abandon. My pussy gets soaking wet as I ride him up and down. I then I push my ass up into the air and Jon lubes my tight ass and his cock. He slowly puts his first few inches into my ass. It feels different, but I'm so turned on that I don't feel it that much. He begins pushing more and more and now he is all the way in my tight ass. Oh my God, it feels amazing. Throughout all this I continue to fuck Craig. With two cocks now securely in me, I start to cum. "Oh god I'm going to cum" I scream. I cum as their cocks pound my pussy and ass.

In time we decide to switch. We would now stand up and I would get fucked like a sandwich. As I'm standing, Jon kind of holds me up and Craig does the same as it's now Craig's turn to fuck me in the ass. (Of course they use condoms and clean up before entering my pussy if previously been in my ass.) It was so different, bizarre, wild and dirty! As I'm cumming I tell them that I want to be their naughty slut who loves to suck and fuck.

Wow, I can feel their cocks bump against eachother from time to time through my flesh. Suddenly the testosterone really kicks in and they get into a competition to see who can fuck me in the hole they're in the hardest and fastest. We are like animals. What fun we are having. The sweat is pouring off our bodies and we are groaning and moaning like wild beasts. Gosh knows how many calories we burning! My pussy is dripping and all the friction felt great.

10. My husband spent over an hour last night playing with my anus. He wants to take me there but I think it's a sin so I say no, but he's so persistent so I agreed to let him play with it as long as he wants, as long as he doesn't take me there with his penis.

Well he now plays with my anus often using his fingers and sex toys. Last night was for the longest time by far.

Last night he sat on chair (we call it "the chair") in the middle of the room and told me to lay over his lap, like I would be if I was getting a spanking. We're both naked. Next to him on the right is small table. On it is what he'll use on me. It has the lube, sex toys (the use of which I don't think is a sin), towel to wipe me and/or himself off with and anything he is going to spank me with like paddles, a strap and sometimes even a hairbrush!

First though, after I was done cleaning up from dinner, we went into the bedroom and I gave him a long massage. As is normal we were both naked and while I straddled him, massaging him, he played with my breasts. I love it when he does that.

Finally it was time for me to use my mouth on his penis so he could have an orgasm. I laid down on my side and sucked away, feeling his cock get harder and harder in my mouth. It wouldn't be long before he filled my mouth with his seed.

We rested for a while then he told me it was time for us to go to the "chair". My husband just loves to play with my asshole. It took me a while to get used to it but now I really enjoy it.

I lay over his lap. He massaged my butt and legs then tells me to spread my legs. He then uses a vibrator on my vagina until I have an orgasm. It was so nice. But that was just the beginning. I then get a spanking with two of the paddles. During the spanking he'd use the vibrator on me again, often I can orgasm from just that but for some reason I couldn't last night. Then it was time for my anus to be played with, and it would be played with for a very long time!

After that we go back to the bedroom for intercourse.

11. My 34th birthday was one I would not forget. My fiancée promised me a special and unusual birthday and that is certainly what I got.

We've been together for almost two years. Our sexual interests have evolved a good deal. One of the things that's developed was our interest in anal sex. Now when we have sex, Jack starts in my pussy and finishes in my ass.

Ok, so after my birthday party, we were alone.

We kissed and cuddled on the couch for a while then Jack told me to go to the bedroom, strip, get on the bed and wait for my birthday surprise, which I did.

As he was about to enter the room he told me to close my eyes. I heard him enter and felt a bunch of stuff get dumped onto the bed in front of me. He said I could open my eyes and low and behold, sitting in front of me, was over a dozen brand new anal sex toys still in their wrappers! Jack told me that they all were going to get used on me tonight!

First I was scared and started to feel a tightness in my stomach, though also a throbbing between my legs. I bet I got wet then and there.

I looked the toys over. There were two anal trainer kits, couple of "lube shooters" to get the lube in all the way, 2 rump shakers, 6 butt plugs of various sizes, a vibrating anal probe, 3 sets of anal beads, all sorts of exotic lubes, a black throbbing anal balloon that gets inserted and inflated to stay securing in an ass, another expandable butt plug, 2 fingered butt plugs, an anal dilator kit and an oversized flesh colored butt plug that looked like trouble.

Well guess what we did nightly for some time! It was a blast, though sometimes I would need a night or two off for my asshole to regroup. After that night Jack would play with my ass with one or more of the anal toys, then we would make love.

Ladies what are you getting for your birthday?

12. You cover my eyes with a blindfold and tell me to bend over the back of the couch so my naked ass is in the air. I hear you moving behind me but don't know what to expect until I feel one of your lubricated fingers probing my tight little hole. You insert another wet finger which I can't help but start fucking. With your free hand you slap my ass hard and tell me to stay still. Then you remove your fingers and I feel another pressure against my hole. It's bigger than your fingers and I realize that it's a butt plug and from the feel of it one of the largest you have ever used on me. I want to pull away but know that wouldn't be right so I brace myself as you slide it in, which you do gently at first until the initial resistance of my muscles has passed, then you push hard so that the full length is in me. I moan again at this intrusion.

I hear a noise and realize that you inserted an inflatable butt plug and now you're inflating it. You inflate it past the point of comfort but I keep quiet. You then attach both of my hands together with handcuffs. You then tie ropes around each of my ankles which spread my legs good and wide, tying each ankle to opposite couch legs so my holes are on display for all to see. I am now immobile with my pussy and asshole sticking out very invitingly, even though my ass is full. Then you turn and leave the room. I am now alone and scared but I've been like this before so I start to feel a familiar tightness in my stomach and that wetness between my legs. I know that you will return and fuck me to your heart's content. Each thrust you make into me will also pound up against the inflated butt plug in me. While you're taking me you will reach down and play with my tits at will. I will cum so hard for you.

13. She said her name was Carla but who knows. She charged me $50 to fuck her in the ass. I never saw signs of STDs on her but again who knows. She would come over to my apartment, strip and jerk me off until I was hard. (Sometimes, unfortunately she would first go into the bathroom and snort cocaine before sex which was really uncool.) After she got me hard she would put a condom on me, lubed me up real good and get on her hands and knees, or elbows and knees. I didn't need to be particularly gentle in taking her in her ass and could slide right in and fuck hard within seconds. She loved it too. She would play with her clit with her hand and/or a vibrator. I'd spank her butt too as she'd start begging for that after a while.

She'd give me up to 20 minutes of ass fucking (I only fucked her in her pussy once but it was too loose and frankly I was pissed she even made me pay money for that.)

If I hadn't cum within 20 minutes, I'd pull out and she would lube my dick up even more and masturbate me to orgasm, which she was really good at actually.

Anyway, I heard she got busted for prostitution and hoped it wasn't anything worse. What sucked was I was afraid that the cops had gotten pictures of me with her or something, which fortunately they hadn't.

Anyway I really miss that tight ass and how much she enjoyed being fucked in it. I've fucked two ladies since but both wouldn't let me fuck their ass, which really sucks.

14. I'm a 36 year old white female that's been fucked in the ass many times. The first two times I was drunk which may be the best way to get acquainted with getting it in the ass.

I have a fuck buddy that loves fucking me in the ass. It was the first time for him and I think he hardly can believe his luck, not only am I a pretty no commitment fuck buddy but I love it up the ass too.

Well he did something the other night that blew me away. He called and told me to clean out my asshole really well (which I did before sex anyway.) He seemed really serious about it so I enemaed and soaped and did all the cleaning I could. Something was going on here as he was never like this. I also had to wonder if he wasn't freaking out in terms of thinking I was a dirty slut or something of that nature. That would be a hassle if I had to find another fuck buddy but doable as I went through dieting hell to get down to a size 6.

Anyway he came over to my place and we had the usual chit chat, watched American Idol and retired to my room when my nosey roommate came home.

Our clothes were off in a jiffy and wow did I ever have a treat, he ate out my asshole, as in with his mouth, and not for a minute or two but for 20-30 minutes!

He tongue fucked me several times throughout it all, often he played with my clit during all this.

I had never had this done to me and after I got over the surprise, I realized how excited I was. Fortunately I had 2 different vibrators within arm's reach and I put them to quick use on and in my pussy. My orgasms were amazing.

Girls if you're into anal sex you've got to experience this. Warning to the guys, tongue fucking an asshole for a long time can really make your tongue sore!

The End

Book #8 - 100 Great Lines To Put in Your Personal Ad

Copyright © 2013

100 Great Lines To Put in Your Personal Ad

Introduction

The lines in this book can be combined with other lines you may think of to make your personal ad all it can be. Some lines in the book might need adapting to best suit you and/or your sex.

TAGLINES: Your short "tagline" is a headline that, perhaps along with your picture, can get readers to further explore your ad. Great taglines are like gold and people have paid hundreds of dollars for them! Now however many are on the Internet for you to see and use.

Remember, people love to laugh. A funny tagline is a big plus.

There is a great deal of material in this book to build quality taglines from. You may also want to take a bit of time and do a web search for "best personal ad taglines" for ideas. Chances are others (including those looking at your ad) haven't seen the tagline already, or have forgotten it if they did.

The Lines

A day not in love is a lost opportunity.

My friends know me as spontaneous, spritely, and upbeat.

I am searching for a beautiful person inside and out.

Are you looking for real love and someone special?

I enjoy thought provoking dialogue.

Together let's seek our destiny.

I hope only to fulfill your every desire. Is that too much to ask?

I love making people happy and to see them smile, even if at times it is at my own expense.

I feel the most pleasure when I know I am doing/enduring something to please another.

I'm looking to learn, not just to play....

I'd like to explore hidden fantasies with you.

I want to be taken to that special place and beyond.

I have the financial and emotional capacity to take care of myself.

Unlike perhaps others here I'm not misrepresenting myself. I know the importance of honesty.

I need to be with someone who has a high self esteem, is confident in themselves and who if they have baggage, knows how to deal with it. I love challenges too so if you dare me I won't hesitate to do it.

I love sex. Rough sex, fun sex, emotional sex... I want you to respect me before and after but during is negotiable.

I want to explore my naughty side,

I'm looking for a friend, confidant and lover.

Like me I'd like you to be thoughtful, attractive, and looking to expand yourself as a person.

I have developed intricate pleasure techniques which can slowly arouse and pleasure beyond imagination.

I think I would describe myself, briefly, as quite a sociable person with a good sense of humor who doesn't take herself too seriously...having said that I believe I am also thoughtful and caring and someone who places great value on good friendships and relationships.

I am loyal, compassionate and respectful of people and animals. People describe me as easy going and good natured.

I have got great plans and goals in my life which I want to achieve.

I'm a contemporary yet spiritual soul in search of his charming, compassionate and caring companion to share this journey of life.

Are you looking for someone to grow with and push things further?

I have a wise mind and younger spirit.

I am an easy going, and loyal friend.

I'm looking forward to a fantastic voyage of a relationship.

I am attracted to someone who enjoys learning and growing.

Are you looking for fun, adventure and a challenge? If so I'm your girl.

I'm a passionate person with interests numerous and diverse.

I am trustworthy, affectionate, passionate, loving and non-judgmental. I am happy with myself and my accomplishments.

I want someone kind, loving, honest, communicative and self-aware. Your developed interest in education, hygiene, aesthetics, style and emotional literacy would make life easier for us. I'd like to find someone interested in building a relationship based on an accomplished life and a win/win attitude.

I am looking for someone who can work themselves deep inside my mind and make me fall to my knees.

Are you looking for someone to make you happy...someone that won't just have sex with you but will make love to you?

We all want to achieve heart pounding serenity.

I am looking for something more than just sex and games. Sure sex is a part of it but I also want someone that I can spend time with. I want the total package.

I want someone that I can go out with, talk with, laugh with, and fall in love with.

Outside of our playtime, I'd like to enjoy a harmony that can grow into a loving, trusting relationship. I enjoy the outdoors and staying healthy, going out on the town from time to time and hanging out at home.

My last relationship ended because we grew in different directions.

I am usually lucky and love life. I would like to find someone like that.

I'm a strong, seductive, passionate woman who is established and knows herself.

I'm well educated and well-travelled. I'm gainfully employed and very independent. I enjoy traveling, good food and wine, the theater and sports.

I'm searching for an open minded man with an adventurous soul and sensual heart. A journey in love is the destination. We still have plenty of time but none to waste! A beautiful world is waiting. Let's enjoy while we can!

I'll laugh at your corny jokes.

I'm a writer and voracious reader. I'm smart, and I like smart people.

Physical attraction leads to animal instincts.

I have a strong passion for the exploration and power of touch in all its forms.

I enjoy knowledge, I like to learn new and exciting things.

I am cosmopolitan and highly educated. I am a baby boomer, in good shape and would like an agemate and a partner who understands mutuality. I am interested in developing a long term relationship.

I am interested in meeting someone who is honest, open and enjoys (his) her kink.

I have very many interests and I'm passionate about all of them! I love movies, literature, music, art, theatre, science... and lots of other things.

I am fun, open-minded, spontaneous and down for raunchy action.

The reason openness is important to me is that it shows that someone accepts themselves.

I'm lively and active and have a well developed sense of humor.

I hope to always be me and take advantage of any opportunities and chances whenever they're thrown at me.

I am totally devoted when in love.

I'm a laid-back, drama-free kind of person.

I want to be late to my own funeral.

Physical play is quite enjoyable but chemistry and a connection is more important.

I like to laugh, I like to have fun.

I believe that love is not what we see but what we do.

I won't ignore you or abandon you. I'm not looking for a secondary relationship.

I have a well developed and dominant sexual identity. I am seeking a man who is a smart, uninhibited, challenging partner.

I consider myself a natural leader, an innovator, a creator. I fight for the best and readily take the risks incumbent with leading a fulfilled, enriched life.

I am a strong, confident thinker, with a secure sense of himself (herself).

I consider myself to be a spontaneous, fun loving person. I work hard, play hard, and enjoy life. I'm a very affectionate and passionate. I like to hold hands and believe it or not cuddle. I believe in treating others the way I would like to be treated. I am looking for someone to grow with spiritually, mentally and physically. I want someone who is not afraid to love and be loved, someone who is affectionate, passionate and good kisser.

I will love you and take good care of you. I am someone who you can trust and believe in, someone who will always want to make you feel happy.

I'm neat and clean both internally and externally.

I want true love and real commitment.

I am looking for something more than just sex and games. There is a balance that is needed since none of us can live in a purely sexual world. Sure sex is an important part of it all but I also want someone that I can spend time with. I want the total package. I want someone I can go out with, talk with, laugh with, and fall in love with.

I want something that will naturally grow and evolve into its own very beautiful story.

I enjoy a great number of things and am very open to experimentation.

I'm interested in your fantasies.

I want to touch your body, your soul, your life.

I still believe that fairytales can come true, it can happen to us...

I live a healthy lifestyle. I am seeking the same.

I am brimming with sexual desire.

I will be looking forward to hear from you and Your wish will always be done...

I am looking for a partner - but I am happy to form a friendship.

Living on earth is expensive...but it does include free trips around the sun.

I eat healthy and workout regularly.

I am an educated, intelligent professional with eclectic tastes in most everything: art, music, food, people, entertainment and travel.

I'm looking for a non-smoker to share my life with in all ways, a friend and companion to travel with, commiserate over bad days and rejoice over good days; a lover and confidant.

Educated, professional and kinky.

I have class and style. I know the value of dressing to impress.

I would love to be able to say "I've finally found you."

I believe that we all have the ability to create or change anything.

I consider myself to be a sharp, crafty, inventive, fun, strong woman who enjoys life more when she's in a relationship.

I'm looking for a like minded man to chat, debate and play with.

I'm not a just fantasist wasting your time.

I am people biased not gender biased.

I am family-oriented and have family values.

I possess confidence but take pride in not being arrogant. I'm persistent but respectful. I have intelligence and charm.

I don't like negative people. We're here to live life not fear it.

I have learned in life that the smallest good deed is better than the grandest good intention. I have high hopes for us.

I am a sharp, crafty, inventive, fun woman who doesn't hate men or hate anyone for that matter.

I enjoy life so much more when I'm in a relationship.

What you are like OUT of bed makes you more desirable for me to want you to take me there.

I like to please as much as be pleased.

I want to discover and explore my limits as well as push them further.

I like intellectual conversations.

My ambition is self-actualisation, to release the potential within.

I'm thoughtful, devoted, industrious, competitive, genuine and trustworthy.

I'm looking to learn and grow, not just to play....

The End

Book #9 - How Women Can Get More Pleasure
from Their Breasts

Author: Michelle Tallia

How Women Can Get More Pleasure
from Their Breasts

The specialized breast massage discussed in this book can give a woman a surprising amount of pleasure. If her lover is unavailable to pleasure her this way women can easily give themselves *Extreme Pleasure Breast Massage*, and it's something women can do to themselves for the rest of their lives.

There are a many positions a woman's body can be in to receive this specialized and very sexually arousing breast massage. For this example though, let's have her sitting up and at least topless. Do note however that as she gets more and more aroused, she'd probably prefer to be naked so one or both of you can access her pubic area with fingers or toys while she's experiencing Extreme Pleasure Breast Massage.

For this position the massager sits behind her with his/her chest up against her back. If it's okay with who is getting the massage, I suggest the massager be naked as many women will lose control at some point when getting Extreme Pleasure Breast Massage and be anxiously reaching behind their lower backs to play with the massager's privates. If a woman has never experienced this type of erotic massage before, she in particular may react with callous abandon.

Before placing yourselves in any of the massage positions, you'll need to have readily available a good supply of quality lotion, massage oil or hair conditioner (yes the stuff you might put on your hair. Thicker hair conditioner is often better and the cheaper brands might work just as well.)

If using lotion, try to use some brand of non-desensitizing lotion. (Most lotion's ingredients include desensitizers to dull the pain of dry skin and other irritations. These desensitizers can at least partially desensitize breasts, thus cutting down on the breast's capacity to provide pleasure.) Baby lotions at dollar stores may be good ones to try but lotions tend to vary by brand. Optimally you want the massaging medium to stay slippery as long as possible and, not cause any irritation of course. Cold lotion/oil/conditioner on breasts can provide an unwelcome jolt so if warming is necessary, warm the lotion/oil/conditioner up ahead of time using the microwave oven, or by setting it in hot water. Make sure the top is loosened somewhat incase it warms up too much and creates steam. (You can also rub together blobs of it in your hands to warm it up.) Always have an ample amount of this massage oil/lotion/hair conditioner nearby as well as small towels to wipe it off of your hands and her breasts after the massage is over.

Put a sizeable glob of massage oil/lotion/conditioner on each of your hands, rubbing it all over the palms of your hands to spread it out, as well as warm it if it's not yet warm. Then put your well lubricated hands on her breasts, *but not yet on her nipples and areolas*. This is because those provide the most pleasure and thus the best is saved for last!

It is so important that the massager make sure to keep his/her massaging hands *very* well lubricated. When the oil or lotion is breaking down the massager will feel stickiness developing. **It is now time to put more massage oil/lotion/conditioner on!** The rule of thumb is that you can't lubricate your hands and her breasts too much!

Also the massager needs to make sure his/her nails and skin of their hands are smooth. Trim and file your fingernails and that kind of thing, to as short and smooth as possible. Otherwise she (the person receiving the massage) might feel them as they rub against her sensitive skin. She can even get hurt by them because as she is in the thongs of ecstasy, she might not realize that they are hurting her, so make sure to watch out for her and take care of this situation.

Typically the massage will provide three levels of pleasure. Massaging the fleshy part of her breast (but not massaging her areolas and nipples) should give her pronounced and very welcome pleasure; of course the faster her breasts are massaged the more pleasure she'll get.

Including her areolas in the massaging will increase her pleasure a lot. But massaging her nipples will really get her going.

Below (and not in order of importance) are suggestions to optimize the breast massage:

* Start from the bottom of her breasts (where the breasts meet her torso) and work your way slowly higher up to just below her

areolas. You can move your hands at varying speeds but typically the faster you massage the more pleasure she'll get.

* Simultaneously circle her boobs with each hand. Start out by using limited pressure on the breasts while utilizing only one finger, then gradually work your way up to utilizing all your fingers. Go clockwise then counterclockwise (or vice-versa.) Remember, *leave her nipples and areolas alone as much as possible until she's practically (or literally) begging for you to massage them.* Sure you will "bump" into them from time to time as you massage around them. Those bumps will give her a delicious taste of what's to come.

* At its base, wrap each hand around a single breast then run your well lubricated hands around and along that breast in a steady spiraling motion up the breasts in the direction of her nipples, until you reach the edge of her areolas. Of course you can go in the opposite direction also (starting from just below her areolas and working your way down to where her boobs meets her torso.)

* Place one hand on the base of one breast; the back of the hand should be facing her head. Put your other hand on the base of her *other* breast, the back of it should be facing her legs. Slide your well lubricated hands from left to right and then vice-versa, across and along both breasts.

* At its base, take each breast in a well lubricated hand and with increasing speed pull up from the base of her breast toward the nipple until your fingers reach the edge of the areolas (or if you're already playing with her areolas and/or nipples, go all the way to her nipples.) Then do the opposite and slide your hands back down from the top of her breasts to the breast's base (where you started from.) Repeat this procedure many, many times.

* Tease her by sliding only your well lubricated, manicured fingertips over her breasts, wiggling your fingers.

* Instead of the above, perhaps for a minute or more, you'd like to start the festivities by teasing her breasts by only briefly touching them here and there using only the tips of your fingers.

* Concentrate your efforts on only one well lubricated breast; wrap both hands around it, kneading it, pulling it and twisting it.

As previously discussed, it's strongly suggested that you take your time before playing with her areolas and then nipples. This is because she will still get a good deal of pleasure from having the 'areola and nipple-less' massage. I for one require that she even beg you to play with her nipples--because as we know this is where the breasts offer the most pleasure.

Before finally massaging her nipples (admittedly you will "bump" into them periodically,) I would suggest waiting until she is already well stimulated. You may stroke her anticipation by whispering in her ear that you're about to play with her nipples, then suddenly do it! She may scream with delight as an orgasm overcomes her.

Playing with her nipples is typically the high point of the massage. She'll likely be getting the most pleasure now. (Again, the faster your well-lubricated fingers move around her nipples, the more pleasure she's likely to get.)

Okay massagers you now have a choice, you can immediately start massaging her nipples fast and hard, driving her crazy, or start massaging them slowly, then progressively massaging them faster and faster until she screams in ecstasy. If you're going to massage them fast immediately, as is the first option, many women will start their orgasm then (if they haven't already.)

Don't forget you can let her use a vibrator on herself as you massage her and thus it's suggested you keep a vibrator within her arm's reach. Believe me she'll find it if it's there.

Because so often the woman you're massaging will get so aroused from all this, that with both hands she'll instinctively reach around her lower back to play with the massager's pubic area. She then will not have a free hand to use the vibrator on herself. (Of course both your hands are busy giving her Extreme Pleasure Breast Massage.) A way to counter this is to secure a vibrator with white medical tape (the type used to hold gauge and cotton to cuts etc.) over her most sexually sensitive pubic area. (Perhaps it would be helpful if she keeps her panties on for extra support.) If you do this, more women will orgasm while you are giving her Extreme Pleasure Breast Massage.

Remember guys her nipples can get tender after orgasm and need to be left alone for at least a bit of time.

As is obvious, ladies, you can give yourself Extreme Pleasure Breast Massage in the privacy of your own bedroom.

After the massage, ladies your breasts tend to become firmer for a while and often they'll feel quite good for hours.

The following is another way of giving this massage, (told from the perspective of the kinky dominant massager.)

I will tell you to stand up and we will go to the bed (if we're not already there.) I will set the bed up so I am sitting with my back against the headboard of the bed and you are laying in front of me face-down on cushions (on the bed) with your head positioned so you can easily suck on my penis and play with my scrotum.

Also I'll put a roughly 3' x 3' sheet of plastic under your upper body to keep the massage lotion/oil/hair conditioner from going on the bed covers.

Perhaps I will also tie your hands together and perhaps then also to the headboard. If I do that though I will make sure there is enough slack in the rope for your hands to still move freely around my penis and scrotum while you suck. If your hands are tied to the headboard, I will be sitting on the rope as my butt will be in-between your bound hands and the headboard which your hands are tied to.

Your breasts will now be positioned, thanks to these cushions, just above the ground. As you suck on my penis, I will generously lubricate (and keep lubricated,) your breasts with some brand of preferably non-desensitizing massaging medium. I will warm the lotion/oil/hair conditioner up ahead of time or rub it in my hands to warm it up, if warming is necessary. I will then massage your breasts. (Many lotions put desensitizers in them to dull the pain of dry skin. These can at least partially desensitize breasts thus cutting down on the breast's capacity to provide pleasure.) I will continue for a long time to massage your lubricated breasts as you suck on my penis. (Remember to always keep the massager's hands well lubricated! The two of you will quickly notice that the nipples respond with the most pleasure from this massage.)

Using a yardstick type implement, I can reach across your back and spank you as you suck. Obviously one should make sure the woman can handle being spanked while sucking. Most can depending on the intensity of the spanking and how hard she's already orgasming.

The End

Legal Notice: In this publication there may be inadvertent inaccuracies including technical inaccuracies, typographical inaccuracies and other possible inaccuracies. The writer and publisher of this publication expressly disclaim all liability for the use or interpretation by others of information contained in this publication and/or listed Web sites. The author, publisher and distributors of this publication hereby disclaim any and all liability for any loss or damage caused by errors or omissions, (should these exist) whether such errors or omissions resulted from negligence, accident, or other causes. If legal advice or other expert assistance is required, the services of a competent professional person in a consultation capacity should be sought. the information contained herein may be subject to varying state and/or local laws or regulations. All users are advised to retain competent counsel to determine what state and/or local laws or regulations may apply to the user's particular business. The Purchaser or Reader of this publication assumes responsibility for the use of these materials and information. Adherence to all applicable laws and regulations, federal, state, and local, governing professional licensing, business practices, advertising, and all other aspects of doing business in the United States or any other jurisdiction is the sole responsibility of the Purchaser or Reader. The Author and Publisher assume no responsibility or liability whatsoever on the behalf of any Purchaser or Reader of these materials. Any perceived slights of specific people or organizations are unintentional. Products, services and websites' content vary with time. Please verify any published information. *eBay is a registered trademark of eBay Inc.

Book 10 - The Absolutely Essential Guide To Buying On eBay

Copyright 2013

The Absolutely Essential Guide To Buying On eBay

Table of Contents

35) Check Cashback and Voucher Websites
36) eBay has trained teachers that could be in your area
37) Join the many eBay Forums
38) eBay Research Tool 1
39) Ebuyeredges.com eBay Research Tool 2
40) Buy Refurbished Products
41) Numerous Other Creative Ways to Find Items to Buy.
42) Order Samples Before Buying If Possible
43) Keywords & Relevancy
44) Perhaps Check Amazon.com's Webpage For The Product
45) Flaws in Items Make Items Less Expensive
46) Payment Options
47) SquareTrade Warranties
48) About Me Page
49) People Selling with 0 Feedback
50) Best Time To End Your Auction
51) Sellers like to Drop Ship When Possible
52) eBay Stores
53) The eBay Store Identity

BUYING ON EBAY

1) Last Minute Bidding Frenzies - Perhaps you've noticed that often there's a bidding frenzy in the last minute of bidding. New bidders may start bidding then in the hope that the previous bidders will not be watching, or can't increase their bid in time. Often however it's because of *Sniping*.

Sniping websites automatically bid on your behalf, often in the last 10ish seconds. Simply sign up, enter an eBay item number and the maximum price you're willing to pay. Hidbid.com and Goofbid.com offer sniping services that place bids for you.

Typically you'll need to give sniping sites your eBay password for them to work (ugh!!) Obviously that is a serious security concern.

There's little protection from eBay if things go wrong when sniping, as you willingly gave your password to a third party. If you do sign up for such a service, never use the same password for eBay as you do for other accounts like bank accounts or email addresses.

2) Second-chance Auction Scams To Beware Of - Unscrupulous people sometimes watch bidders in high-dollar auctions and try to take unsuspecting buyer's money after an auction ends.

The scheme, known as a *Second-chance Auction Scam*, is just one of many types of Internet auction frauds the *Internet Crime Complaint Center,* or *IC3* hears about.

Second-chance scammers wait until auctions end and then offer bidders that lost a phony second chance to purchase the item -- usually through a wire transfer service. Beware!

3) Misspelled Item Search Tool - Typojoe.com, Goofbid.com, Bargainchecker.com and Fatfingers.co.uk, Baycrazy.com - There are many items listed on eBay every day that have misspelled words in the title. It's unfortunate for the seller but chances are good those listings will not come up well in eBay's search engine (because misspelling causes keyword search problems) and thus not bring the seller top dollar.

4) *Special Bidding Tip* - Often sellers start auctions at .99 cents, (or at least under a dollar) hoping a bidding war will erupt. Many items go unspotted, staying at this super-low price (99 cents).

LastminuteAuction.com hunts for eBay auctions due to finish within an hour but where the price still is very low.

With these items in particular, double-check delivery charges, as some sellers hope to recoup costs by charging a little extra (though eBay's now set maximum delivery charges for many categories).

5) *Don't Forget About Facebook Marketplace* - *Facebook Marketplace* is a force to be reckoned with. Also sellers often are open to haggling. Just log on to your account at Facebook and search for "Marketplace". It's also worth checking to see if there's any local Facebook selling groups in your area.

6) *Nigerian Type Scam for Paying EBay Auctions* - These unscrupulous people want to pay with a money order that they often claim to already have handy. Often it's for more than the purchase amount. He writes to ask if the seller would be "honest enough" (or something of that nature) to send him the extra cash along with the item. (However he might just try to only buy the item with it and not ask for extra cash.) Unfortunately the money order can look okay but it is counterfeit. They particularly like the *Buy It Now* feature.

7) *Set Long-term Alerts For Rare Items* - If you want something very specific or hard to find, set a "favorite search" and eBay will email each time a seller lists your desired item.

Simply type a product in eBay's search bar, such as "silver dollar", and click "Save Search". Be as specific as possible for the most accurate results. When (and if) someone lists one, you're alerted with an email.

8) Don't Assume eBay's the Cheapest Place To Get Your Item - Many people assume that if it's on eBay, it's automatically the least expensive place to get it, but that's often not the case. Perhaps you'd also like to use *shopbots* (shopping robots) that check numerous Internet retailers to find the best price. Megashopbot.com is one. Type into a search engine "shopping comparison sites".

The same rule applies when buying used merchandise. Check used marketplaces on Amazon.com and Play.com - you may even get it for free on Freecycle or Freegle.

9) How To Check the eBay Going Rate For an Item - There's a quick way to check an eBay product's average price. Enter the item into the search box and click "Completed listings". What will come up is a list of prices that similar auctions have already settled on. After that, sort it by "Price: lowest first". If the price is red, it means no one bought it. Green means it sold. Figure out the average price.

10) eBay has banned the selling of intangible items, and that includes curses! - Among the items that were prohibited as of August 30, 2012, are "advice; spells; curses; hexing; conjuring; magic; prayers; blessing services; magic potions; healing sessions; work from home businesses and information; wholesale lists, and drop shop lists."

11) Haggling on eBay Can Pay Off - There's nothing wrong with asking for a discount, even if the listing doesn't have the "Make offer" indication. Haggling works best on *Buy It Now* listings, or auctions with a high start price and no bids. Also you'll likely do better if you haggle as the auction is coming to a close as the seller could start feeling more desperate.

To contact the seller, click on the seller's nickname then "Contact seller". If you're polite, you'll likely get further. Blunt requests such as "dude, how about $15?" likely won't work out as well. Remember the seller is likely going to lose money doing this so no point in being annoying.

Once you've arranged a deal, try to keep the transaction within eBay. Ask the seller to add (or change) a Buy It Now price. That way you don't lose the usual eBay buyer protection privileges.

12) Other Things to Do To Exploit Sellers' Screw-ups - Some sellers make basic mistakes, leavings goods going for bargain money. "

As well as spelling boo-boos, another error is to leave out key details such as shoe size, dress brand, saying a console's a Wii when the photo shows a Xbox. At this point, many buyers give up on that listing as it's "too much hassle".

So contact the seller to fill in the gaps, but don't ask the question via the item's listing page, (because that way, when the seller replies, eBay lets them add their reply to the main listing, so it's no longer your secret.)

Instead, ask the question via the seller's About Me page. (Make it clear which item you're talking about). This way they might not bother with the extra hassle of adding it to the listing, if so you'll be the only one in the know.

Also the seller might not realize how underpriced the item he/she actually has is.

13) Tool to Track Down Crazy EBay Auction End Times - Listings that finish at anti-social times often get fewer bids, thus sell for less. To locate auctions that finish when fewer people are around to bid on them, use BayCrazy's *Crazy End Time* search. (A lot more on the best times to end your auction later on.)

Check out their auto-bidding tools if you don't want to spend all that time in front of the computer bidding at odd times. Other BayCrazy.com tools include "unwanted gift" and "ending now" searches.   www.baycrazy.com/search.php?page=nightowl (Baycrazy offers other eBay related opportunities also.)

14) Search Descriptions as Well as Titles - eBay automatically searches seller's titles for results that include your specified keywords. If you're not getting the results you want, try also searching the item's *description* too. (To do this go to Advanced Search.) For example, imagine you were searching for a REI Jacket. Unfortunately the seller may be selling one but only put "Ski Jacket" in the title however he mentioned "REI" in the description. Include description in your search and then it should then come up.

15) Search Using eBay Boolean Logic - If a seller could describe an item in different ways, you can make an eBay search for several different ways of describing it at once. Just place "((" at the beginning and enter different phrases individually enclosed by quotation marks, then followed by commas.

So for example, type... (("fishing tackle", "hook", "reel" ...and it will simultaneously bring up listings that contain the words "fishing tackle", "hook" and/or "reel".

16) Add A Few Extra Cents to Your Bid - When bidding, if you enter a "maximum bid", eBay makes automatic bids on your behalf up to your maximum bid.

Don't enter a round number. For example, if a coat is currently selling for $20, and the most you're willing to pay for it is $25, enter a maximum bid of $25.24. If someone tries to outbid you by entering the round number of $25, they will receive an outbid notice. eBay will go your bid, even though it's just 24 cents more.

It's worth being aware of bid increments, the steps by which prices rise. For a list, see *eBay's Bid Increments* guides by looking that up in a search engine.

17) Be Somewhat Skeptical of Feedback - eBay buyers and sellers have a feedback rating that acts as a useful guide to previous seller's opinion's of them. As a guideline, look for a seller with more than 98% positive feedback and a high feedback score of at least 30. Also ensure you read their feedback from their *selling*, not just their *buying*. (To see their feedback, click on their username.)

18) Seller with Zero Feedback Could be Cause For Concern - Think twice before purchasing expensive items from a seller with zero feedback.

Remember feedback's useful but not infallible. One thing to watch for is traders selling a number of cheap things for $1ish each to build their feedback, and then suddenly listing items costing hundreds each.

19) Check to Make Sure You're Bidding on the Actual Item - Sometimes you assume you're bidding for an item on eBay (or any auction site,) when all that's actually being sold is a link to another site selling what you want. People are not suppose to be able to sell these on eBay anymore but they can fall through the cracks.

Always read the whole description in detail before bidding. Often the catch is hidden in the text at the end – an attempt to protect the seller from any recourse.

20) The Before Bidding, Contact Me Request - Beware of it - It's a red flag if a seller writes "Before bidding, contact me" then asks for a money transfer. Thieves who hijack actual eBay accounts might use this tactic.

21) Paying with Western Union or MoneyGram - Beware of it - Always be worried if you're asked to pay by an instant money transfer service such as Western Union or MoneyGram. Instant money transfer payments often cannot be traced and are highly popular with thieves.

22) Sneakily Find Underpriced Buy It Nows - Feel free to hunt for *Buy It Now* bargains also. Perhaps the seller under-values their item making their price a good deal.

To look for them, in advanced search, select a category you're interested in and filter it to show *Buy It Now* items only.

23) Always Complain within 45 Days - Under eBay's buyer protection program, 45 days is the most number of days you have to open a case if you're unhappy with your purchase. (There are some exceptions such as tickets for events that are months away.) Read more on eBay's protection policy.
http://pages.ebay.com/help/policies/buyer-protection.html#conditions1

Under eBay's own Buyer Protection rules, buyers are eligible for a refund if the item's "not as described", meaning it didn't match the seller's description. http://pages.ebay.com/coverage/index.html

24) Pay by PayPal - Avoid sending checks and try not to use use money orders. It's much harder for scammers to disappear with your cash when you use eBay's online payment system, PayPal. As this way you're covered by eBay's Buyer Protection program. If an item is faulty, counterfeit or non-existent, you are far more likely to get a refund.

25) Outbid? Here's a Way To Maybe Get It After all - Missed out on a desired item by pennies? Don't give up hope. As every seller knows, sales sometimes don't materialize when buyers change their minds or can't come up with the dough. Because of that feel free to send a friendly message such as: "Hi, I've been looking for this poster for years and just saw your finished auction. Please let me know if the sale doesn't come through or if you have another to sell."

They may send you a *Second-chance Offer*, which are sent out by sellers to unsuccessful bidders if the winner fails to pay up. Ask them to relist the item at an agreed *Buy It Now* price.

26) Know Your Consumer Rights - When buying from a person who makes or sells goods for resale on eBay you often have the same rights as when buying in person from a shop that does the same. This means your goods must be of satisfactory quality and as described.

With private sellers it's buyer beware. Buyers' only rights under law are that the product is fairly described and the owner has the right to sell it.

Under eBay's own Buyer Protection rules, buyers are eligible for a refund if the item is "not as described", meaning it doesn't match the seller's description.

27) Beware of All The Fakes - While eBay has a 'flag and remove' policy to help identify fakes, still plenty fall through the cracks.

If you're buying big-name brands, do your research first. Carefully check sellers' feedback and post on the forums to get others' opinions. Be especially wary of overseas sellers or branded items that seem especially cheap.

The more *unprofessional* the photos, likely the better. Thieves often take professional photos from the brands' sites. Legitimate sellers typically take photos of items at home that might not come out as well.

28) Think Twice Before You Give A Seller Negative Feedback - Of course, negative feedback is often justified but have a heart, don't leave negative or even *neutral* feedback without first trying to work the issue out with the seller. Most sellers are good folks who will try to help, particularly, as it can mean a lot to their business to stay in your good graces.

Remember eBay users can view the feedback you've left for others, and if you leave a significant amount of negative feedback, they may well decide you're too high of a risk to sell to.

29) Add An Item You're Interested in to eBay's "Watch List" - Want to keep track of an item without bidding on it? eBay lets you add items to a "Watch List", so you can relax knowing you'll get an email reminder significantly before the auction ends. To watch an item, just click the *"add to watch list"* link in the upper part of the item's eBay webpage.

30) Avoid Private Purchasing If Possible - Sellers may suggest you do a deal outside eBay for a cheaper price. If you do you'll likely have less protection if things go bad. You won't be able to leave negative feedback and you won't be protected by eBay's Buyer Protection Plan.

31) Think Safety When Picking Up An Item In Person - The usual precautions apply. If you get to their door and the seller's holding a butcher knife, now's the time to run.

32) Think International - There's bargains to be had on overseas eBay sites. To include foreign auctions in search results, click "worldwide" for location.

Still can't find what you want? Another option is buying directly from *international* (foreign) eBay sites. The main ones are USA, Canada, Australia, Germany, France and Spain - there's a full list at the bottom of eBay's homepage. Make sure that the item reads *"Shipping to: worldwide"* before bidding as some international sellers only do business with their country's buyers.

Always factor in postage and if applicable, custom fees. Remember that return postage fees could be hefty.

Also what kind of credit card protections will there be? You're often still protected by eBay and PayPal's buyer protections (if you use PayPal), but it's worth investigating. Type in "buyer protection" in PayPal.

33) Don't Forget The Online Classified Ads - Again, let's not assume that because it's on eBay, that's where you'll get the best price for an item. Unfortunately that's often just not the case (though you might be better protected if you buy it on eBay, or at least using PayPal.).) Type "top classified ad sites" or something of that nature, into search engines. There's also *Freecycle* and *Freegle*. (Those two sites offer free stuff. freecycle.org and ilovefreegle.org.)

Remember, anyone can post on these classified ad sites. If someone asks you to pay by MoneyGram or Western Union, as always be concerned. It's a bad way to pay.

34) Check Other Auction Sites Also - There are other auction sites that can be found through search engines. If you're searching for something specific, it's also worth adding it to your search. *Auctionlotwatch*.com is a useful shopbot for online auctions. Search for an item and it crawls the big auction sites for you.

35) Check Cashback and Voucher Websites - Check cashback websites to see if there's money back available on your eBay purchase. Type into search engines: "cashback and voucher sites".

Cashback sites give you a cut of their proceeds by setting you up with product and/or service providers.

36) eBay has trained teachers that could be in your area. Also see eBay University. Check out:
http://pages.ebay.com/sellerinformation/howtosell/university.html

37) *Join the many eBay Forums* - Ask questions about anything, selling, buying etc. Great information is posted already and could be of use. Work together as a team. Find eBay and other auction forums by looking those up in search engines. EBay hosts forums.
http://forums.ebay.com/category/Ebay-Discussion-Boards/2001

38) eBay Research Tool 1 - To help in your research about items, you can go to eBay's top sellers webpage and see what's selling best.

39) Ebuyeredges.com eBay Research Tool 2 - You can use Ebuyers (www.ebuyersedge.com) to just search eBay for items as well as set up a saved eBay search (or a number of them). You'll get alerted with an e-mail when a matching item is listed.

40) Buy Refurbished Products - Refurbished products fall somewhere in between new and used products. Refurbished products are not new, but often they aren't significantly used either. Sometimes a customer buys the product and for whatever reason, returns it for a refund. The item is then returned to the manufacturer, given an inspection, repaired as necessary and sold as refurbished.

There are various ways an item can become refurbished. The packaging of an item can be damaged during shipping. In that case the item is sent back to the seller/manufacturer.

Refurbished items usually come with manufacturer's warranties. Although sometimes the warranties that come with refurbished items are for a shorter period of time, the products are usually in very good condition.

Items that have a slight defect or flaw, like a scratch or mechanical flaw, might be returned to the manufacturer. The manufacturer repairs the items, repackages them and marks them refurbished.

Demonstration units are also considered refurbished, but generally that's when they're returned to the manufacturer, inspected and repackaged.
Brand new overstock items can also be marked refurbished. Sometimes it's a situation where only the packaging of an item is opened or damaged. It's re-packaged or even just closed up and marked as refurbished.

Refurbished Products Advantages:

1. Refurbished products are significantly cheaper than new products. They also come with warranties, boxes and everything else new products come with.

2. Selling refurbished products is often profitable, even though refurbished products cost significantly less than new products. On eBay (and at other places) refurbished products can sell for the same price as new ones. (Many people buy refurbished products thinking they're buying new ones.)

3. Refurbished products are sometimes new! When you buy a lot of refurbished products they might actually be overstock items or factory overruns. In that case you would be buying new products at a fraction of the price.

Refurbished Products Disadvantages:

1. Refurbished is not new, even though refurbished products can be exactly the same as new ones, people simply prefer new items.

2. Refurbished products are sometimes previous year's models. If you're selling electronics or computers it could bring the selling prices down.

41) Numerous Other Creative Ways to Find Items to Buy.

a) YELLOWPAGES.COM - www.yellowpages.com. Try this first. Yellowpages.com can find specialized suppliers in your area. Type in "wholesale" into the search box and you will be given a bunch of subdirectories to further explore. Make sure the search is based on a location near you. Next type "wholesale directory" or "wholesale directories" into search engines.

When searching also try inputting keywords such as overstock, salvage, surplus, liquidation, auction, refurbished, refurb, supplier, closeout, wholesale, etc.

b) BUY FROM AN ACTUAL EBAY SELLER. Buy multiple items and get a discount. That discount could be your margin of profit.

c) BUY WHOLESALE LOTS FROM EBAY AND RESALE THEM - Go to eBay and search for "wholesale lot". If you buy a big lot, you could find you profit best by individually selling the items in the big lot.

d) PERHAPS SELL DIGITAL COUPONS. You should be able to get them for free. As of this writing, people are posting that coupons sell well on eBay. If you're selling coupons, you need to mention that your auction is for the time you spend finding, assembling (sorting) and sending the coupons to the buyer rather than selling the actual coupons themselves. It's illegal to sell coupons themselves and that's why auctions say the payment is for the time to gather and sort them. Still you're providing a service as it can take time to find good coupons and first folks need to know where to look. Important, cover yourself legally .

e) BUY FROM LIQUIDATION COMPANIES - A liquidator is someone that buys overruns from big retailers (Sears, K-mart, Wal-Mart etc.) at a fraction of the wholesale price. Sometimes big stores can't sell everything they have. The stuff they couldn't sell needs to be gotten rid of as soon as possible to make room for new products. This is where liquidation companies come in. They buy the overruns, often at a fraction of the wholesale price. When a liquidation company buys a couple of truckloads full of overruns, the next thing it must do is sell these overruns ASAP to make room for more overruns. Since the liquidator must get rid of the products as soon as possible, the products are sold at cheap prices and often in bulk. Perhaps there are liquidator stores in your town what would make you a deal and you wouldn't necessarily have to buy in bulk. Perhaps you can find something there to individually sell on eBay. The smaller and lighter it is the better.

f) You can sell peoples' houses, cars, boats, or even jewelry collections. Just look in the for sale listings of your local newspaper and look at all of the great stuff for sale that would sell on eBay. Call up the owners of the items advertised in the newspaper and offer to sell the stuff for them. Looking for stuff in newspapers is great because the people that are using a newspaper to sell something probably know little about eBay and are desperate to get rid of the stuff they're advertising. These people are also the ones that are willing to lower the price and haggle, and that is great because the lower the price they're willing to let the item go for, the more profit you can make by selling their stuff.

g) RUNNING ADS TO FIND MERCHANDISE - You can run ads in print media and/or post what you're looking for in Internet forums with something like "I will buy your stuff". As previously noted, if you are going to use this method you'll need to pick a used product that keeps its value well. If you're going to use this method you should buy things like jewelry and watches, antiques and other things that appreciate with age.

A previous seller's success story was selling old collectable Apple computers. This is a type of item that some people have laying around in the basement or attic, and will likely never use again. They're more than happy to unload it and get a little money for it at the same time. But on eBay it was a whole new ballgame. There are thousands of people who collect old collectable computers.

42) Order Samples Before Buying If Possible - This is a particularly good tip if you don't have a chance to inspect and see the products you're ordering in person. Many people starting out on eBay make the mistake of placing a big order before actually seeing what they're ordering. By ordering samples you'll be able to test not only the quality of the products you're ordering but the service, communication and legitimacy of the company you're ordering from. If you're thinking of selling designer clothing on eBay, be extra careful. There is a lot of fake (counterfeit) clothing being sold on the Internet. Remember the pictures on the supplier's website may look real, but that doesn't mean they will be sending you what's in the picture.

If you find a great deal but the "supplier" won't allow any sample orders and wants you to pay through an untraceable method, be wary.

43) Keywords & Relevancy - Make sure the brand name of what you're buying is in the title! If you're buying a Champion Portable Generator, your eBay search should include the make and model number, in this case "New Champion 42431 Portable Generator, 1500 Watt". The listing title typically is a short, abbreviated description of the item.

The name of the product in the title has to do with the search results (keywords). If people want to buy a portable generator they may search "portable generator, generator, Champion, Champion portable generator," etc. You want to be checking in as many search results as possible.

44) Perhaps Check Amazon.com's Webpage For The Product - If you want other people's opinions on a product you're interested in that's being sold on eBay, you might want to check for the product on Amazon.com's website as Amazon posts product feedback from customers where eBay doesn't.

45) Flaws in Items Make Items Less Expensive - There may be a flaw in an item you're looking for, or in an item that you could be interested in. It could make it a better deal. Put "flaw" related words in the eBay's search engine, as well as the name of the item and see what comes up.

46) Payment Options - You should be offered several different choices of payment. Most pay through PayPal, (PayPal is owned by eBay,) so make sure you get a PayPal account (www.PayPal.com). Of course, not everyone who buys items on eBay prefers PayPal, some may prefer Western union's Bidpay or another payment system. If you're interested in buying from international auction sites (including eBay international sites) you might be interested in StormPay as it can be used by people in some countries where PayPal is not used, or is as popular. For your free StormPay account go to: stormpay.com.

Wire Transfers - Unscrupulous overseas buyers prefer these as they're not as traceable. It's preferable not to use them.

47) SquareTrade Warranties - If applicable to what you're buying, you might want to get a SquareTrade warranty for the item you got at www.squaretrade.com. Keep the purchase information as they conveniently don't send you that, likely in hopes that you lose it and can't use the warranty. www.squaretrade.com/seller-faq

48) About Me Page - If interested in buying something, you might want to look at the seller's *About Me page* . The *About Me page* is often overlooked by many eBay sellers (and buyers.) While having the free About Me page likely will not dramatically make it easier for you to buy, it can help if you have good things to say about yourself and a nice picture.

49) People Selling with 0 Feedback Ratings - Having a good to great feedback rating is so important as you know. If the seller has no feedback, it could be cause for concern. Many sellers refuse letting members with 0 feedback even bid on their auctions. Getting a negative feedback from somebody that unpredictable is simply a risk we don't want to take.

50) Best Time To End Your Auction - The best time for an auction to close (end) is in the evenings and on weekends as that's when most people are on the Internet for that type of activity! An auction ending any other time might not go as high, which could be a good thing for you! If you're selling you'll want to make sure that when your auction is closing (ending), when everyone that's interested in the item is available to bid on it. The mornings are the times that the eBay website gets the least visitors (as people are more often sleeping or working.)

If you live in the Eastern Time Zone, list your auction between 9pm-11pm, Central Time Zone list between 8-10pm, Mountain Time Zone between 7-9pm, and for the Pacific Time Zone list between 6-8pm. This will give you the biggest exposure at the end of your auction. The debate is out as to what day your auction should end on. Some sellers report that Tuesday, Wednesday and Thursday are best. Other sellers report that Saturday and Sunday are best.

There are a few exceptions though. For example, some business products sell best during weekdays and during work hours. Obviously this is because people are usually ordering those types of products at work, for work. Studies have shown that a listing that ends at peak hours can attract up to 25% more bids than one that ends in non-peak hours. Listing your auctions at optimal times is one of the easiest ways to attract more bids.

To end the auction in the evenings, you'll need to put the item for sale in the evening (*or use listing software [soon to be discussed] to do it for you*) as eBay considers each day to have a length of 24 hours.

Note, it's eBay's practice that when someone's auction is ending, that listing shows up higher on keyword search results (which is a good thing for them!)

51) Sellers like to Drop Ship When Possible - With drop shipping all the seller has to do is list items up for auction and when they sell, contact the supplier, who ships the products from their factory, straight to the customer. In theory drop shipping is a good way to go, but it could offer problems. What happens when an item sells and the supplier sends them to the wrong addresses? What happens when an item sells and the supplier is out of stock? In those cases your reputation suffers. If using drop shipping make sure there is good communication between the seller and supplier (drop shipper.) The seller should also have some products in stock in case the supplier runs out by the time the auction closes.

52) eBay Stores - eBay stores can be great if you're looking for a number of items to buy (or sell). To have an eBay Store, first you'll need to reach the minimum number of feedbacks required (10). Most PowerSellers (special higher volume eBay sellers with a closer relationship to eBay) have eBay stores. Store sellers can see an increase in profit of up to 25% in the first three months of opening the store (according to eBay). Having an eBay Store can save a substantial amount of money in listing fees and let sellers items in a fixed price format as well as selling via auctions. Also items can be listed for a much longer time and stored in an inventory list for 30, 60, 90, 120 days and even "Good till Cancelled". You can feature links to other auctions in all your listings by utilizing a cross promotion tool. There are also bonuses like your own search engine and monthly reports from eBay featuring statistics and dada about your sales in the past month.

An eBay store also gives a location to go to. It gives a base of operation, and a place where repeat customers can come back to. Customers will be able to bookmark and return to the store, and it may also be indexed in the major search engines. So if you're selling silver dollars, and someone does a BING search for silver dollars, your eBay store may appear in the results along with the usual online retail websites! Obviously this can increase your traffic greatly, and likewise boost your sales.

53) *The eBay Store Identity* - Ideally the eBay store should look different from its competition. One can use the design templates eBay offers, but perhaps it's best to use original graphics. Fortunately eBay Stores are customizable.

The End

www.ingramcontent.com/pod-product-compliance
Lightning Source LLC
Chambersburg PA
CBHW070900290526
45795CB00001B/187